YOGA-AYURVEDA MIRACLE

(*Ancient Wisdom Spawns World Medical Traditions*)

M. K. Agarwal Ph.D., M. D.

Director of Research Emeritus

Founder Aum Ayurvedics

A. K. Sharma, B.A.M.S.

(Ayurvedacharya)

Artha Ayurveda Center, India

A Theoretical and Practical Guide to Wellness

First published by Dog Ear Publishing
4010 W. 86th Street, Ste H
Indianapolis, IN 46268
www.dogearpublishing.net

ISBN: 978-145750-339-9

This book is printed on acid-free paper.

Printed in the United States of America

TO

ALMA MATER

honor

scholarship

uncompromising integrity

Acknowledgments

The research conducted for this book stems from my lifelong quest to assign correct historical perspective to the Vedic-Buddhist patrimony of ancient Bharata that was usurped by the successive aliens who invaded India over the past 1000 years and more. After having freely stolen the insights gained by the ancient sages of Bharata since the beginning of recorded antiquity, the invaders despised the very peoples whose material and intellectual riches were usurped by armed might, mutilation, murder, torture, deliberate mistranslations, omissions and the like. Thanks are due to my alma mater for opening the door to inquiry and instilling in me a sense of balance, justice, objectivity and righteousness.

I am indebted to the staff and facilities of libraries at Bryn Mawr College, the TriCollege collections and their Inter library loan services, as also the libraries at the University of Pennsylvania, Columbia University, and many others. Some of the rare books were made available to me by various sources in India where several leading experts in Sanskrit provided valuable insights into the message hidden behind the apparently specious poetry of Vedic aphorisms. For illustrations, I am thankful to the patient enterprise of many who went through the trouble of understanding technical terms for a nonspecialist public. Many colleagues at the University of Paris, despite their own hectic schedule, gave me their invaluable advice, ideas, criticisms, and suggestions for improvement.

Finally, the sheer abundance of the unsurpassed patrimony of ancient Bharata, both in terms of quantity and quality, is so rich that my journey into the past cannot be completed within one lifetime. However, I have decided to stop here and share my experience with those who seek truth in place of bias, inquiry in place of dogmatism, serendipity in place of insipid logic, wisdom in place of ignorance, self analysis in place of condemnation, and introspection in place of indoctrination… The present era has been called the 'Asia Century' so I hope that my effort will contribute to the revival of those peoples and traditions that have either been destroyed by the intolerance of the invaders, or gathering dust as they lie buried in the forgotten shelves of human endeavor.

Sattyameva Jayate

M. K. Agarwal   February 2011.

PREFACE

The quest for health and longevity is as old as the history of the human race. Ayurveda-Yoga disciplines took birth in the cradle of the Indus-Sarasvati Civilization (ISC), some 5000 years BC, where wealth was generated by agriculture as well as maritime and terrestrial trade, such that peace and plenty permitted the great Rishis in *tapovans* to meditate upon human welfare. The secrets revealed to them by nature were later recorded in the Vedic literature that far surpasses all other ancient knowledge in quantity, quality and antiquity. All medical and mathematical traditions of the Vedic world can be traced to these Vedas which were further expanded into Vedangas, Upanishads and more specialized literature. The ISC was oriented towards the well being of its people and ushered in 'The Age Cleanliness' in the form of planned cities replete with covered drains and toilets. Concurrently, highly advanced surgical techniques, well developed Ayurvedic pharmacoepia, and the discipline of Yoga, assured a disease-free life which is said to have spanned several hundred years for some individuals. All of these accomplishments of the ISC were freely globalized through trade, wandering scholars, and monks, in the zealous spirit of *krinvantum vishvamaryam* (civilizing the whole world). More dissemination of the Vedic-Buddhist patrimony took place through the great Universities of Taxila and Nalanada where students came from as far away as Greece, Egypt, the present Middle East, China, and the South East Asia. Indeed, the Ayurvedic theory of humors was to form the backbone of health care around the globe until the 17th century. Ayurveda itself underwent significant change with the arrival of Buddhism when products of animal origin were gradually discarded in favor of metals and herbs.

The 'Greek miracle', 600 BC on, grew out of the knowledge they received from the ISC as Greece had no scientific, cultural or literary tradition prior to this era. In fact, Greek-speaking invaders consisted of seminomadic tribes that penetrated the Balkans around 2000 BC, founded the stronghold of Mycenae around 1600 BC, and raided Troy (Ilium) probably around 1230 BC. In the 9th-10th century BC, Homer (Homeros means hostage), took up the oral tradition of the last four centuries and transformed the rape of Troy into a war of honor in the epics of Iliad and Odyssey. Thereafter, Greece entered a dark age until 800 BC when land hunger saw the rise of Greek colonies in Europe, Asia and North Africa. Consequently, Greek miracle was a product of borrowed knowledge, as the Greeks themselves acknowledged. In fact, the medical tradition assigned to the Hippocrates in Greece was an idea invented primarily by the British to assert white racial superiority though medicine in Greece was a handmaiden of philosophers whose medical theories were absurd, to say the least. Indeed, there was no written source anywhere in the world for the development of medical discipline, in contrast to the vast Vedic literature.

Similarly, the Bedouin Arabs were a nomadic people who looked upon arable land as a benevolent deity whereas their high god was a moon deity by whose silver white light they grazed their land and whose benevolence cooled the air. Poetry was the principal medium for the expression of Bedouin, Arab collective memory and spiritual life, though some of the tribes in the south were more advanced. With the expansion of Islam into Asia, translations of Ayurveda texts became Yunani medicine, while translated Vedic sciences took the names of their Muslim translators to be passed off as Arabic heritage. Indeed, the culture of vanquished lands and peoples became Arab culture.

The scientific and medical supremacy of the ISC-Buddhist-Jain tradition remained unchallenged until the 12th century CE when invading Turks sacked Nalanda and translated the Vedic-Buddhist patrimony into their own medium. These translated texts formed the backbone of the European universities, founded only as of the 11th century CE. Europeans not only exterminated peoples and cultures around the globe, they freely copied from the traditions of the enslaved peoples, while false translations by white colonial masters were planted to further ridicule the colored subjects. In reality, until the 17th century CE Europeans had no accomplishments of their own because the Biblical Pentateuch of 800 BC, which is just Jewish history, was supposed to possess all knowledge required by man. Although European imperialism has excercized an absolute monopoly on words like progress, civilization, and the like, and calls itself the society of tomorrow, it is in fact a society of yesterday as it adopts practices that it had previously rejected due its own religious dogmatism and false vanity.

This book is meant to set the record straight by providing a total perspective, in contrast to the hundreds of specialized books these past few years. First of all, it traces the origin of the Ayurveda-Yoga tradition to the oldest and the most extensive philosophical ideation in the Vedas. In Samkhya philosophy, the *sattvic* mind knows no disease which stem from desire when the mind becomes mired in its limitations and sense objects. The sister disciplines of Ayurveda and Yoga were developed to reverse the Samkhya theory of evolution such that the microcosm (man) may once again find oneness with the macrocosm (God). Second, it relates various traditions of Yoga to the New Age Therapies and the manner in which the former have provided the conceptual basis for the latter. Third, it contrasts the symptomatic western medicine with the holistic care in the diagnosis and treatment of afflictions prevalent in the contemporary society. Finally, it reveals that Ayurveda influenced the primitive medical practices in other parts of the world, and permitted the development of modern European medicine from 18th century on, not the other way around. Also included are practical tips for a balanced life at home through daily and seasonal routines of Yoga, Ayurveda, nutrition, and time tested recipies. The political entity known as India from the period of the British era on was initially part of the ISC-Baloch-Persian cultural zone and known by various names in the antiquity. From *Sindhu* the Greeks derived the word *Indos* leading to India whereas the Persians pronounced it as *Hindu* and hence *Hindustan*; other names include *Bharata, Jambudvipa, Melhuaa, Aryavarta, Aryadesha, Mlecchadesa, Brhamdasa desa* and *Ophir.* As the term 'India' reeks of the era of colonial imperialism, when the Vedic-Buddhist patrimony was denounced, the word Bharata has been used here as much as possible.

CONTENTS

1.

Geopolitical Setting

The Ice Age ended nearly 15,000 years ago such that by 8000 BC the freshwater locked in the Himalayan and Tibetan glaciers was unleashed into great perennial rivers: Sindhu (Indus), Sutlej, Sarasvati (now dry), Yamuna and Ganga in the North West India, and Brahmaputra, Irrawady/Mekong in the east. Of these, the Sarasvati was the mightiest river during the prime Rigvedic age (8000-2500 BC), but went extinct around 1900 BC. Rigveda pays hommage:

Foremost mother, foremost of rivers, foremost of goddesses, Saravsati
We are, as 'twer, of no repute and dear Mother, give thou us reknown.
In thee, Sarasvati divine, all generations have their stars.
Be, glad with Sunahotra's sons: O Goddess grant us progeny.

The Sarasvati hymn in Rigveda venerates the number seven which occurs constantly in Yoga and Ayurveda (chapter 9).

She hath spread us beyond all foes, beyond her Sisters,
Holy One. As Surya spendeth out the days,
Yea, she most dear amid dear streams, Seven-sistered,
Graciously inclined. Sarasvati hath earned our praise.
Guard us from hate Sarasvati, she who hath filled the
Realms of earth. And that wide tract, the firmament!
Seven-sistered, sprung from threefold source, Five
Tribes prosper, she must be invoked in every deed of might.

The Indus has been invoked in Rigveda as Sindhu:

Flashing and whitely gleaming in her mightiness
She moves along her ample volumes through the realms

Most active of the active Sindhu unrestrained
Like a dappled mare, beautiful, fair to see.

Unconquered Sindhu, most efficacious of all the efficacious,
Speckled like a mare, beautiful as a handsome woman.

The seven great rivers in the **Sapta Sindhu** region, called *hapta hindu* by the Persians, ushered the Neolithic around 10000-8000 BC where the Indus-Sarasvati Civilization (ISC) took shape as the most ancient phase of what is now called Indian culture (Figure 1). Spread over some 2.5 million square kilometers, an area the size of Western Europe, it was the largest of the four ancient civilizations of Egypt, Mesopotamia, India and China. Rich alluvial desposits in the flat valleys of these mighty rivers permitted the development of agricultural settlements at an unprecednted scale. According to Dr. B. Sasisekaran, *"The carbon dating of 7,500 BC obtained for the wooden piece recovered from the Indus sites changes the earlier held view that the first cities appeared on the horizon around 3,500 BC"*. Conclusive evidence is present at Mehragarh to refute the reductionist dogma that techniques of food production "somehow diffused" in a unidirectional manner, from the culturally advanced west to the Near East and then into a "primitive" south Asia.

The ISC people **pioneered the cultivation of wheat, barley, cotton and rice** for the first time in the world, **transformed cotton into thread, and invented the spinning wheel** to weave the cotton thread into cloth. This ideation is no less important than the control of fire to assure survival and the use of cotton spun in the ISC preceded its introduction into other parts of the world by some 2000 years. Similarly, the **domesticated fowl** was perhaps one of the greatest achievements of Harappans, as all domestic species descend from the wild Indian jungle fowl, and it later spread to Egypt, and China via Burma. The ISC peoples kept several breeds of dogs and possibly house cats, **domesticated sheep, goat, cattle, horse and camels** by 4500-4000 BC; **silk worms** were introduced by 2500 BC. **Water buffalo**, too, was known in Harappa and arrived in China comparatively late.Mining, **metallurgy** and chemical engineering,were all highly developed, as evident by technical ingenuity in smelting, compounding, alloying, casting, and moulding by the lost wax process. The beginning **of iron smelting** in India may well be placed as early as the sixteenth century BC. Pliny refers to *"swords of good quality made of Indian steel"* called 'Damascus blades'. Persians considered that Indian swords were the best and termed them *Jawabi Hind*. Both the Indus Script and Egyptian hieroglyphs may date back to 3200 BC to form *"the earliest system of writing in the world"*. Colonizers from the Indus valley took **urbaniza-**

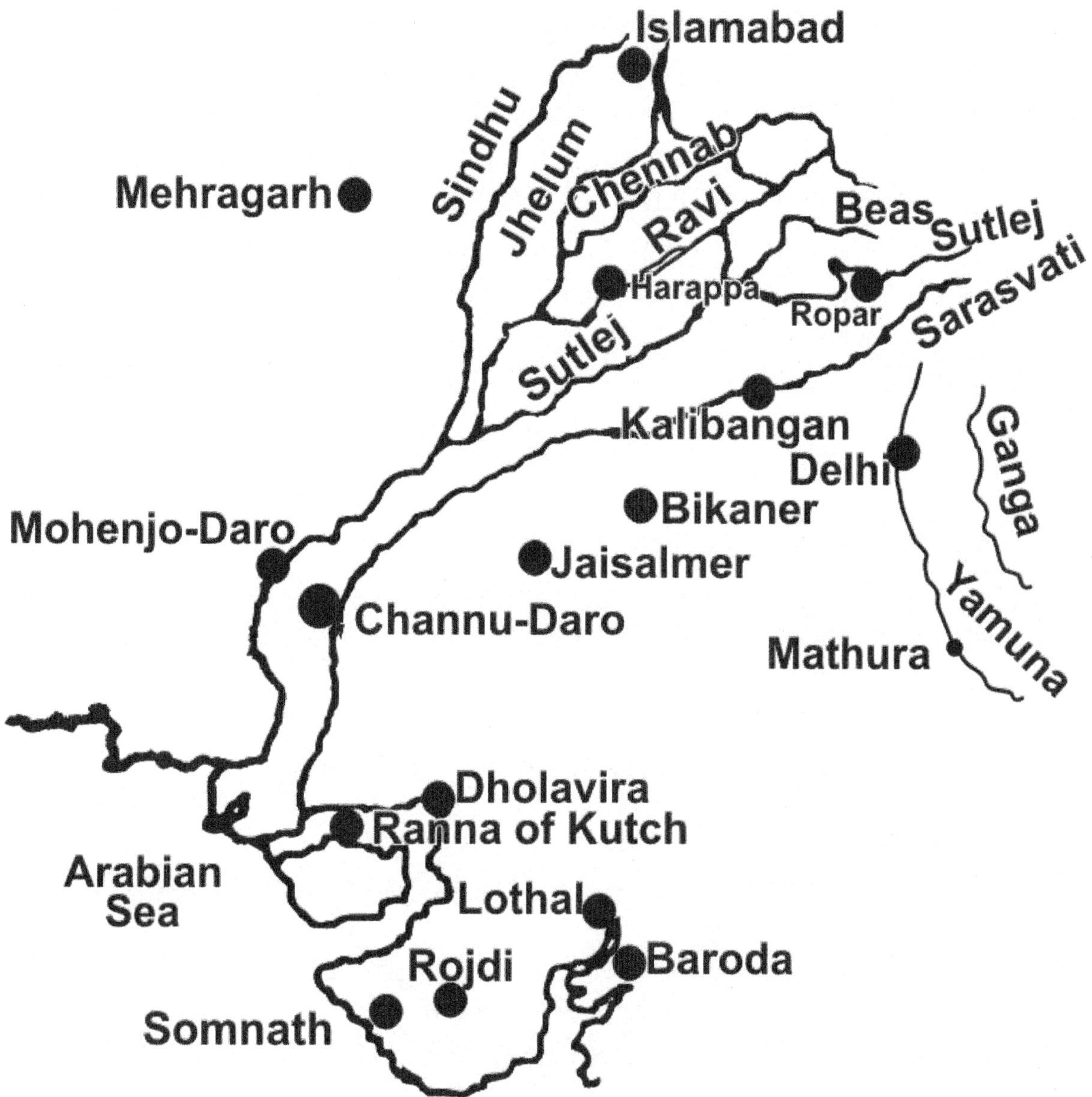

Figure 1. The sapta sindhu region along with some of the major urban centers of the Indus Sarasvati Civilization.

tion and writing to Mesopotamia, rather than the other way around and *"there is a direct continuity from the Harappan script down to Brahmi"*, as delineated by SP Gupta.

The ISC ruling elite controlled **vast trade networks** with Central Asia, Oman, Mesopotamia, Arabia, Persia, Gulf, Mesopotamia, Iran, Turkemania, Uzbekistan, Afghanistan, south-west India, and SE Asia (Figure 2). The Middle Eastern Interaction Sphere **(MEIS)** was based upon revolution in maritime technology that permitted the "Dilmun" trade between Mel-hun or Meluhha (ISC) and Dilmun (Bahrain), so mentioned in the records of Sargon of Akkad (2334-2279 BC), as well as Magan (Oman). The whole area was interconnected by nomads, traders, thinkers, transporters, bards, messengers and craftspeople. Mesopotamian texts refer to objects imported from Meluhha and Dilmun and by 2000 BC, the ISC also traded with Bactria-Margiana Archaeological Complex **(BMAC).** Trade later expanded to the **SE Asia and China** by sea and the Silk Road, the **Greek** world and the **Roman** Empire. Authors such as Pliny lament the drain of gold on Roman treasury for the import of luxury items manufactured in Bharata and transshipped through that region after import from China and SE Asia. Colin Renfrew highlights the fact that there existed a civilization in Europe before the rise of Egypt and Mesopotamia and which was connected with the Vedic civilization. Gold thus poured into India from all directions and the situation remained so until destroyed by the colonial powers.

It is in this context of abundance, prosperity and plenty that great Rishis meditated upon them-selves and the world around them to secure the meaning of existence. In their superconscious state,

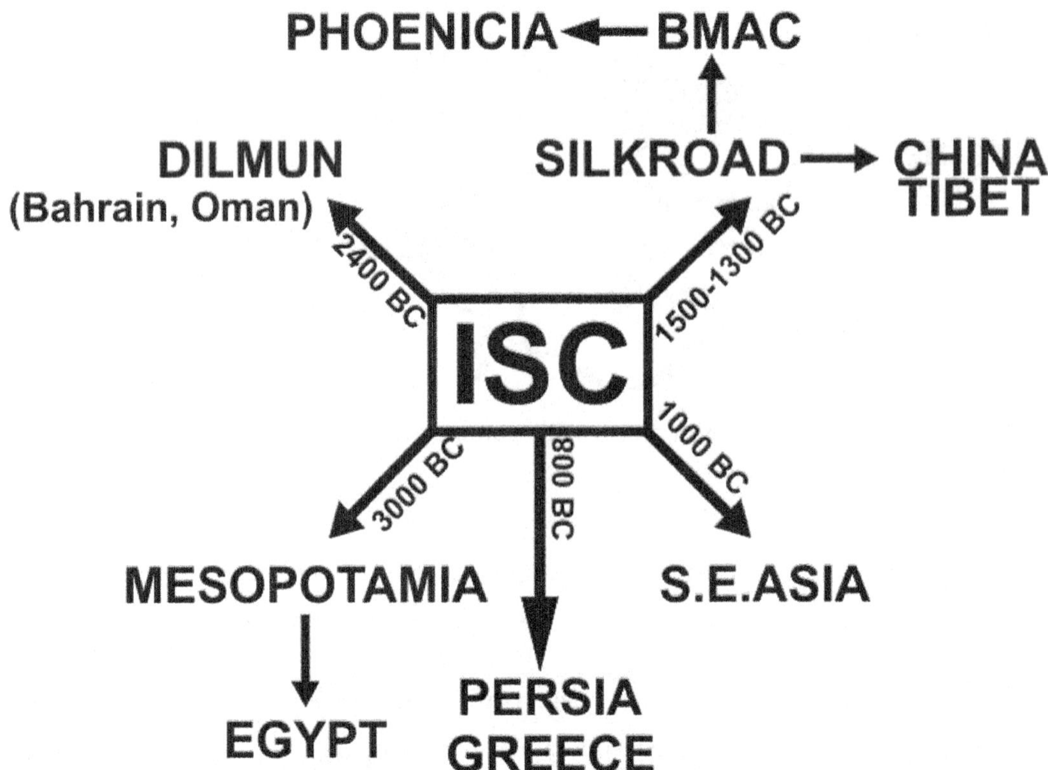

Figure 2. Maritime and terrestrial trade links of the Indus Sarasvati Civilization; all dates are approximate.

they heard the voices of nature revealing her secrets of various sciences and medicine, later recorded in the Vedas (Rigveda is dated 1700 BC and 3200 BC, respectively, by the reductionists and nationalists). The ISC was oriented towards the **well being of its peole**, not on the erection of towering monuments to the kings, gods and priests as in Egypt, Mesopotamia and the Middle East. Mathematics permitted the development of cities like Harappa and Monhenjo-Daro where 20,000-80,000 inhabitants lived behind massive defense wall, in some places 13 feet thick and 13 feet high, made out of **baked brick,** as opposed to the sun-baked bricks of Mesopotamia. A centralized state government took shape in the bronze age of the mature Harappa phase 3200-2500 BC with planned citadels, monumental public buildings, seals, and the very first use of weights and measures. An elaborate water management system ushered in the **"Age of Cleanliness"** in the form **of toilets, sewers, baths, lavatories, covered drains and bath rooms**. Although Mohenjodaro received only 13 centimeters of rain every year, elaborate drainage removed the effluent away from the houses, below ground, safely out of the way and out of sight, in brick lined channels that prevented contamination of the city and the surroundings. The world had to wait 2000 years before Romans could come up with an efficient drainage system and that too was limited to upper class neighborhoods. Ritual purification by water, bathing at dawn and before principal meals, washing of hand and teeth before and after meals, all took shape during the Indus age and continue to this day. Indeed, The Great Bath at Mohenjo-Daro personified personal hygiene for the very first time in the human history.

In contrast, **Christianity** throughout its history appears to have emphasized the grace-giving quality of **dirt and filth.** The Church favored a literal interpretation of the aphorism by Jesus *"but to eat with unwashen hands defileth not the man"*, and forbade hand washing altogether. The Rule of the Christ Church at Canterbury stipulated:

> *"The use of baths shall be offered to the sick as often as it is necessary; to the healthy and especially to the youths, it shall not be so readily conceded".*

The Spanish Christians issued orders:

> *"...for the reformation of Moriscos neither themselves, nor their women, nor any other persons, should be permitted to wash or bathe themselves either at home or elsewhere; and that all their bathing houses should be pulled down and destroyed".*

This practice has not yet entered into the contemporary western society such that the WHO spots on TV constantly remind audiences to wash their hands to stem Swine flu and other communicable diseases.

The basic rituals of the Vedic hindus have been documented on ISC seals like the Pashupati, Yogic posture, ProtoShiva, and mother goddess from 5000 BC on in Baluchistan all of which continued later as worship of Aditi and of natural forces like fire, water, trees, nagas, etc. The sacredness of fire as energy, purity and life giving sun were later on detailed in *Sulba Sutras* to perform public *yajnas* or sacrifices. Vedic medicine was both preventive and curative; the physician was supposed also to examine the food, water, woods, and the environment. It has been rightly observed: "*The people in Mehrgarh tradition (ca 7000 BC) are the people of India today*". Man's **first known trip to the dentist** apparently took place some 7000 to 9,000 years ago at the Mehragarh, the oldest Stone Age complex in the Indus River valley (*New York Times, April 5, 2006*), as evident by drilled molars from a sample of 300 individuals. David Frayer, professor of anthropology at the University of Kansas concludes: "*This is certainly the first case of drilling a person's teeth…But even more significant, this practice lasted some 1,500 years and was a tradition at this site. It wasn't a sporadic event.*" Most of the drilling was done on the chewing surfaces of the molars, probably using a flint point attached to a bow that made a high-speed drill. Concentric ridges carved by the drilling device were found inside the holes.

This rich land with its vast resources, unparalleled tolerance to socio-cultural pluralism, a tradition of unsurpassed ideation, and humanity, welcomed the needy from the world over and shared its accomplishments freely with peoples living in regions that bridged Central Asia to the Far East. The ancient literature of the land far surpassed that of Greece at the time of Alexander's conquest, as noted partly by Alexander Dow in history of India published in 1768 CE, who pointed out that the authentic history of Hindus went back farther than that of any other nation. Tagore observed:

> "*To know my country, one has to travel to that age when she realized her soul and thus transcended her physical boundaries, when she revealed being in a radiant magnanimity which illuminated the eastern horizon, making her rercognized as her own by those in alien shores who were awakened into a surprise of life…*"

Bharata was far more advanced, civilized and literate than England and the rest of Europe until the arrival of Patriarchal religions. Muhammad bin Qasim invaded Sind in the eigth century, while Baluchistan, Afghanistan and Persia, traditionally under Hindu influence, had been Islamicized and were to become launching pads for attacks on Bharata. Mahmud of Ghazni marched into the Gangetic plain after defeating Jayapala in 1001 CE, entered Delhi 1018 CE, destroyed Mathura temples, seized Kannauj in 1018 CE; the destruction of Somnath temple, the kingdom of Candellas in Bundelkhand, cities and temples of Kanyakubja were to follow. The world hegemony of Vedic sciences and medicine was finally over when Nalanda University was sacked by the Turk **Bakhtiyar Khalji** in 1193 CE. Despite all this destruction, under the Moghuls, India was still a magnificent empire rich in gold and precious stones, manufacturing fine muslins and exporting them to the west, while peasants enjoyed a high standard of living.

Indeed, people during the middle ages in **England toiled in a state of perpetual misery and impoverishment**. Around 90% of the population lived in rural areas and worked on the land, going hungry during the frequent food shortages. Begging was common and the nation's ten thousand vagabonds were the terror of the land. Patricide, matricide, fratricide etc were practiced as well, while the living fought for the scarce resources. **Disease epidemics** were frequent and The Black Death still broke out periodically, as did pneumonia, influenza and something unpleasant called "the sweat". Life expactancy stood at just thirty eight years. The vast majority of the English people was illiterate, superstitious and believed in magic; the discontent of communities often boiled over into witch hunts. **Adultery, prostitution and sexual slavery** were the way of life to procure basic necessities, particularly in great urban centers like London. While Victorian moralists preached sexual ideals, red light districts flourished in the second half of the 19th century. Every city had its red light district, possibly as a reaction to middle class ethics which attempted to dictate morality to all classes while reinforcing class distinctions. The works of fiction during the Victorian period include: The Lustful Turk (1828), Rosa Fielding (1876), The Romance of Lust (1870's), The Anatomy Experiences of a Surgeon (1881) and Randiana (1884). They underline the contrast between the public language of Victorian life and literature, and that of sex and pornography. It reveals the discrepancy which existed in the society between openly professed ideals and secretly harbored wishes or secretly practiced vices. Steven Marcus has this to say:

"During the 18th century, the English higher social classes were thought of throughout Europe as the grossest and coarsest of their species. When they ate, they gluttonized; when they drank they swilled; their sports and games were bloody and brutal. Some of these habits persisted through the 19th century. Sexuality was cut off from the rest of life into an insulated sphere. For every warning against masturbation issued by the official voice of culture, another work of pornography was published; for every cautionary statement against sexual excess, pornography represented copulation in excelsis; for every assertion about the delicacy and frigidity of respectable women made by the official culture, pornography represented legions of maenads, universes of palpitating females; for every effort nmade by the official culture to minimize the importance of sexuality, pornography cried out — or whispered - that it was the only thing in the world of any importance at all. Extreme deprivation spurred Pornotopia with its immense, supine, female form, and an enormous erect penis as the supernatural object of Creator and

Destroyer. It could only have been written by men who at some point in their lives had been starved - Sade took the matter to its logical conclusion".

London streets were a veritable barnyard:

"The angle of the street named as leading out of the Strand was dark of a night and a favorite place for doxies to go relieve their bladders...I have seen at night women do it openly in the gutters of the Strand...in the particular street I have seen them pissing almost in rows...Indeed the pissing in all bye streets of the Strand was continuous..."

Strand was of course the place to **pick up children** who did not call themselves whores but who embraced it to treat themselves to "sausage rolls, meat pies and pastries", and to take care of siblings who were locked up during the day in a room without fire and food. Chruchyards were also pressed into service for all such pursuits:

"We when boys, and when youths years later, had laid in wait to see nursemaids and their little charges turn up among the tombs to ease themselves...and there we were laying in copulation, with the dead all around us; another living creature might that moment have been begotten, in its turn to eat, drink, fuck, die, be buried, and rot".

It is this European miasma that set out to 'civilize' the world, particularly India. The British East India Company (EIC) was given official sanction on 31 December 1599 by Queen Elisabeth I, and during 1708-1815 CE the EIC destroyed Dutch, French and Portuguese power and reduced Mughal emperor to a puppet. Lord McCauley in his speech of Feb 2, 1835 CE, to the British Parliament observed:

"I have travelled across the length and breadth of India and I have not seen one person who is a beggar, who is a thief. Such wealth I have seen in this country, such high moral values, people of such caliber, that I do not think we would ever conquer this country, unless we break the very backbone of this nation, which is her spiritual and cultural heritage, and, therefore, I propose that we replace her old and ancient education system, her culture, for if the Indians think that all that is foreign and English is good and greater than their own, they will lose their self-esteem, their native self-culture and they will become what we want them, a truly dominated nation".

The British recognized that they could not stay in India without a local fifth column to support them so Thomas Babbington Macaulay, who was Chairman of the Education Board, was sought to set up an educational system modeled along British lines that would also serve to undermine the Hindu tradition as well as the conversion of Hindus to Christianity. His idea was to create an **English educated elite that would repudiate its traditions and collaborate with the British**. In 1835 CE, Macaulay affirmed:

"We must at present do our best to form a class who may be interpreters between us and the millions whom we govern; a class of persons, Indian in blood and color, but English in taste, in opinions, in morals, and in intellect…and to render them by degrees fit vehicles for conveying knowledge to the great mass of the population".

Macaulay admitted in 1835 CE to having:

"…no knowledge of either Sanskrit or Arabic" yet, he argued, *"that all the historical information which has been collected from all the books written in Sanskrit language is less valuable than what may be found in the most paltry abridgements used at preparatory schools in England".*

Macaulay' s condemnation included everything: Indian epics, Hindu philosophies, arts and crafts that adorned Indian buildings, Ayurveda, and traditions of peoples civilized and cultivated by all arts of polished life while the Europeans were yet in the woods. He observed:

"The question now before us is simply whether, when it is in our power to teach this language, we shall teach languages in which by universal confession there are no books on any subject which deserve to be compared to our own; whether, when we can teach European science, we shall teach systems which by universal confession whenever they differ from those of Europe differ for the worse; and whether, when we can patronize sound philosophy and true history, we shall countenance at the public expense medical doctrines which would disgrace an English farrier, astronomy which would move laughter in girls at an English boarding school, history abounding in kings thirty feet high and reigns 30,000 years long, and geography made up of seas of treacle and seas of butter".

While serving as chairman of the Education Board in India, Macaulay wrote to his father:

"Our English schools are flourishing wonderfully. The effect of this education on the Hindus is prodigious. ……. It is my belief that if our plans of education are followed up, there will not be a single idolator among the respectable classes in Bengal thirty years hence. And this will be effected without any efforts to proselytize, without the smallest interference with religious liberty, by natural operation of knowledge and reflection. I heartily rejoice in the project."

Macaulay wanted someone who would interpret Indian scriptures in such a way that the **newly educated elite would prefer New Testament over their own cultural heritage** as devout Christians believed that the spread of their faith justified all means. He found an impoverished young German Vedic scholar by the name of Friedrich Max Muller who had never been to India but who was willing to undertake the arduous task. Max Muller was promised 10,000 pounds if he could **translate *Rigveda* in such a way as to destroy the belief of the Hindus in Vedas.** This began his work "Sacred Books of the East" but Muller was given only 3000 pounds by the EIC. Max Muller came to England, married an English woman, and developed the two race theory of Cushite-Hamite Negro, and Japhetite or Caucasian, Indians whose darker complexion was caused by the climate. This was later expanded into the Aryan Invasion model and Julian Huxley, one of the leading biologists of the century, wrote as far back as 1939 CE:

> *"In 1848 CE the young German scholar Friedrich Max Muller (1823-1900) settled in Oxford, where he remained for the rest of his life. ... About 1853 CE he introduced into the English language the unlucky term Aryan as applied to a large group of language".*

In 1854 CE, Muller wrote to the Duke of Argyle, then acting Secretary of State for India: *"The ancient religion of India is doomed. And if Christianity does not take its place, whose fault will it be".*

Writing to his wife in 1866 CE Muller observed:

> *"This edition of mine and the translation of Veda will hereafter tell to a great extent on the fate of India and on the growth of millions of souls in that country. It is the root of their religion and to show them what that root is, I feel sure, is the only way of uprooting all that has sprung from it during the last three thousand years".*

H. T. Colebrook remarked:

> *"The British were more cunning at the game than the Portuguese, careful to show respect for Indian religions. Yet they sneered at the pagans behind their back, educated the Indian elite in British-run schools, or at Eton and Cambridge - which, if it did not guarantee conversion to Christianity, resulted in lapsed Hinduism, agnosticism, or an intellectual humanism. In India, Anglo indoctrination produced a generation of "brown sahibs" who looked down on the religion of the masses, the opium of the people. Such is the power of colonization that a whole generation must pass before the paralyzing spell wears off."*

During the colonial era, a handful of Europeans controlled the world resources and peoples at the point of a gun, but had no past scientific or cultural accomplishments to boast of, most of which could largely be ascribed to the Asians, particulalry the ISC. After the 1857 CE uprising, the EIC transferred its domain of India to the British Crown which proclaimed: *"no greater blessing may be conferred upon the native inhabitants of India than the extension of British authority influence and power"*. The British were at pains to stress that they were engaged in a ***"noble mission of ruling a lesser people for their own good"***. The British defined their task as:

> *'the introduction of the essential parts of European civilization into a country densely peopled, grossly ignorant, steeped in idolatrous superstition, unenergetic, fatalistic, indifferent to what we regard as the evils of life and preferring the response of submitting to them to the trouble of encountering and trying to remove them'.*

The British Club soon emerged as the nucleus of white society and Mayo wrote to his Lieutenant Governor of Punjab in 1870 CE *"Teach your subordinates that we are all British gentlemen engaged in the magnificient work of governing an inferior race"*.

Language is the raiment in which man clothes his thought, and the one reacts upon the other – the thought upon the language and vice versa. Sir Rashbehary Ghose (1911 CE) remarked:

> *"Education must have its roots deep down in national sentiment and tradition…We are the heirs of an ancient civilization…In our curriculum therefore, Hindu ethics and metaphysics will occupy a foremost place, the Western system being used only for purposes of contrast and illustration"*.

Tagore enjoined (1919 CE): *"For India to force herself along European lines of growth would not make her Europe, but only a distorted India… When the great European countries found their individual languages, then only the true federation of cultures became possible in the West"*.

In their enthusiasm for things of the West, despising their own vernacular, and rejecting their own classical languages, the **educated Bengalis in early 20th century lost their Indian individuality**. They regarded Sanskrit, Persian and Arabic with supreme contempt *"barbarous, wholesome, unfashionable"*. The ancient scriptures were discredited, Vedas and Upanishads were sealed books and the whole religious literature was an endless void.

> *"Intemperate drinking, and licentiousness of thought, taste and character were fearfully rampant. Infidelity, indifference to religion and point blank atheism were ublushingly professed"*.

Jitendralal Banerji (1921 CE) realized that English education only *"helps to rivet the fetters of our servitude"*.

Sir Charles Eliott summarized thus:

> *"Scant justice is done to India's position in the world by those European histories which recount the exploits of her invaders and leave the impression that her own people were a feeble, dreamy folk…But such military or commercial invasions are insignificant compared with the spread of Indian thought…"*

Gavin and Frost noted:

> *"The original, Victorian translations of Indian texts are highly biased. Not only did they translate many feminine names as masculine, they also could not comprehend that sexual symbolism was meant to serve as metaphor for spiritual truths. In a time when even table legs had*

to be covered (literally by cloth and socially by euphemism), and even the glimpse of an ankle was pornographic, those translators went to one extreme or the other. They either gasped in lewd astonishment over the forbidden writing of the Kama Sutra, or suppressed anything vaguely sexual".

There seems to be little doubt that if the British had not undertaken the civilizing mission in India, the latter would have been freer, more prosperous, far more advanced in science, arts, and all that make life worth living. Unfortunately, the **"History taught today was written by the English to glorify the British rule and virtues and treats Indian past with contempt. It is an apology for and panegyrics of British rule"**. Time has come to shatter the mental shackles imposed by the colonial masters and to reclaim the patrimony that rightfully belongs to the native peoples and cultures around the globe.

2.

Myths and Legends

The quest for healing has always preoccupied the human subject. The cave paintings discovered in Lascaux, France, radiocarbon-dated to13, 000-25,000 BC, depict medicinal herbs in the personal effects of an "ice man", apparently used to treat intestinal parasites. Anthropologists have theorized that animals evolved a tendency to seek out specific plants in response to illness. Indigenous healers often claim to have learned by observing sick animals that nibbled bitter herbs which they would normally avoid. Field biologists have corroborated these hypotheses by observing chimpanzees, chickens, sheep and butterflies, such that **sick animals tend to forage plants rich in secondary metabolites**, such as tannins and alkaloids. Since these phytochemicals often have antiviral, antibacterial, antifungal and antihelminthic properties, a plausible case can be made for self-medication by animals in the wild. Lowland gorillas take 90% of their diet from the fruits of *Aframomum melegueta*, a relative of the ginger plant, that is a potent antimicrobial and apparently keeps shigellosis and similar infections at bay. While some birds select nesting material rich in antimicrobial agents to protect their young, many animals have developed digestive systems especially adapted to cope with a number of plant toxins. For example, the koala can live on the leaves and shoots of Eucalyptus, a plant that is dangerous to most animals. People on all continents have used hundreds of thousands of indigenous plants for treatment of ailments since prehistoric times. The use of herbs and spices in cuisine developed partly as a response to the threat of food-borne pathogens. In the tropics, where pathogens are the most abundant, recipes are highly spiced, particularly with herbs endowed with potent antimicrobial activity. In all cultures vegetables are spiced less than meat, presumably because they are more resistant to spoilage.

The birth of Vedic Medicine has been envisioned thus:

"A scourge fell upon the universe and the disquieted gods came to Vishnu, the father, to ask his advice. In reply, he declared that it was necessary to obtain Amrita, the drink of Immortality, and for this purpose the Ocean of Milk must be stirred up. Therefore, for the time

being, the demons and gods forgot their quarrels and became united in the undertaking of this enormous work.

The great serpent Vasuki coiled himself around the mountain Mandara and the gods and demons, seizing the monster by the head, made him turn the mountain on the back of Vishu himself who had become transformed into an enormous turtle and had sunk to the bottom of the Ocean of Milk.

They labored a long time, and the demons, nearest to the head of the serpent, were permanently blackened by the toxic vapors exhaled from the serpent's head. But finally the work was accomplished and then a moon, a wonderful tree, and a sacred cow came forth from the Ocean of Milk, representing the goddess of Love, Wine, and Beauty, and last of all the physician Dhanvatanri arose dressed in a white robe and holding in his hand the cup of Amrita".

On account of his pity for the mortals, Dhanvatari became reincarnate on earth as a prince of Benares and dictated to Sushruta, the son of the warrior-sage Vishvamitra, the principles of Ayurveda which stem from the antiquity of the Vedic traditions. Sushruta is believed to have transmitted the knowledge to Divodasa, the King of Benares and an incarnation of Dhanvantari.

The **oldest surgical tradition is traced to Jivaka** whose mother came out of a mango flower which was plucked by a *Brahmin;* she later became the famous courtesan Amrapali whose hand was sought concurrently by seven kings. While the kings were deliberating, Bimbisara consorted with her and a son was duly born bearing in his hands a bag full of acupuncture needles. When the new born child was exposed in a public street, Abhaya, the son of Bimbisara from another Queen, adopted him and gave him the name K'iju (Jiavaka). This same account is also found in Buddhist sources. The king wished to make Jivaka his heir but the latter renounced the throne in favor of his elder brother Abhaya and turned to study medicine at Taxila. Jivaka turned to Atri, surnamed Pingula, and spent seven years there as his servant. At the end of this period, Pingula asked Jivaka to find a plant that did not have a medicinal value but he could find none. Pingula declared:

"Go! You now have in your possession the science of medicine. I am the first among those in all Jambudvipa in possession of this art, and after my death you are my worthy successor".

The legend then adds:

"Of the herbs of this world there was not one which could not be employed by him; of the dieseaes of this world there was not one he could not cure".

In the book of plants, the tree King Physician (Bhaisa Jyaraja) could, from outside, illuminate the interior of the human body (like an X-ray). Through Bhaisa Jyaraj, Jivaka lighted up the inside of the body of a girl and took out five hundred worms; the five hundred ounces of gold he received as compensation he gave to Pingla. Through this device, Jivaka could see the displaced liver of a child and performed a laparotomy; this operation earned him five hundred ounces of gold which he gave to his mother. Jivaka also resected the volvulus of intestine which was creating cachexia and emaciation in a man; he now received 200,000 ounces of gold which he gave over to Pingala. When King Bimbisara suffered from an anal fistula, Jivaka cured it as well and the king ordered his five hundred harem wives to deliver all their jewelry which Jivaka refused so he was elevated to the dignity of physician to the harem and member of the congregation (of Buddha). The text of Trehitaka describes how Jivaka cured the wife of a noted person in the kingdom of Saketa and received four hundred thousand ounces of gold, servants, chariots and horses all of which he offered to Abhaya. Jivaka performed memorable **caesarian operations**, as also **craniotomy** for the extirpation of animalcule, for which the rich patient offered one hundred thousand gold coins each to Jivaka and his King. He cured Tathagata of chronic constipation and Jivaka begged that priests from then on be allowed to wear simple lay clothes such that people rivalled with each other in donating clothes to the monks. When Jiavka died, all plants mourned him, saying that henceforth men would employ them without discernment and from their unsuccessful results they would accuse the plants of not being divine.

In another tradition, it is believed that the Ayurvedic knowledge of Brahma passed, successively, from his son Daksha to the Ashvin brothers, and finally to Indra who gave it to Atreya, the author of the fifth book of Atharvaveda. Atreya passed his knowledge down to his students Agnivesha, Bhela, Jatukarna, Parasara, Ksirapani and Harita. Charaka is supposed to have received knowledge directly from Indra, via a Rishi. Ashvins are the doctors of gods and presiding deities of Ayurveda. Ashvin twins are divine horsemen in Rigveda, sons of Saranya, a goddess of the clouds and wife of Surya in his form as Vivasvat. Ashvin gods are also portrayed to symbolize the sunrise and sunset, appearing in the sky before the dawn in a golden chariot, bringing treasures to men and averting misfortune and sickness. They can be compared with the Dioscuri (the twins Castor and Pollux) of Greco-Roman mythology. They are called Nasatya "kind, helpful" in the Rigveda; later, Nasatya is the name of one twin, while the other is called Dasra ("enlightened, giving"). By popular etymology, the name *nasatya* was analyzed as *na* plus *asatya* "not untrue"="true".

In the epic *Mahabharata*, King Pandu's wife Madri is granted a son by each of the two Ashvin gods and bears the twins Nakula and Sahadeva who, along with the sons of Kunti, are known as the Pandavas. To each one of them is assigned the number 7 and to the pair the number 14. Ashvini is the name of an asterism in Vedic astronomy, later identified with the mother of the Ashvins. This asterism forms the first of the 27 asterisms that constitute the zodiac in Vedic astronomy. This star is identified as Hamal, the brightest star in the constellation of Aries (Alpha Arietis). The Ashvins are mentioned 376 times in Rigveda, with 57 hymns specifically dedicated to them: 1.3, 1.22, 1.34, 1.46-47, 1.112, 1.116-120, 1.157-158, 1.180-184, 2.20, 3.58, 4.43-45, 5.73-78, 6.62-63, 7.67-74 8.5, 8.8-10, 8.22, 8.26, 8.35, 8.57, 8.73, 8.85-87 10.24, 10.39-41, 10.143.

3.

Chronological History

Ayurveda is made up of two Sanskrit words: *Ayu* which means life and *Veda* which means knowledge, meaning the science of life, or longevity. To know about life is Ayurveda whose aim was a disease-free life span of one hundred years. **Holism** (Greek *holos*) means *all, entire, total,* and stands for the idea that all the properties of a given system (biological, chemical, social, economic, mental, etc.) cannot be determined or explained by the sum of its component parts alone. Instead, the system as a whole determines in an important way how the parts behave. The general principle of holism was summarized thus by Aristotle in *Metaphysics*: *"The whole is more than the sum of its parts"*. Thus Ayurveda becomes the oldest systems of health care dealing with **both the preventive and curative** aspects of life in a most comprehensive way, in close similarity to the WHO's concept of health in the modern era. This probably makes it the earliest medical science having a positive concept of health to be achieved through a blending of physical, mental, social moral and spiritual welfare. By **contrast, reductionism,** sometimes seen as the opposite of holism, postulates that a complex system can be explained by the *reduction* into its fundamental parts. Essentially, chemistry is reducible to physics, biology is reducible to chemistry and physics, psychology and sociology are reducible to biology, etc. Holism may also be contrasted with atomism.

In the original Vedic system, guru Rishis chalked out the entire course of life for their *shishyas* (students), aged 8-20. Such Vedic gurus included Bhargava, Bhardwaja, Gautama, Shandilya and Vashishta. Sage Atreya, a student of Bharadwaja, lived in the Punchanada area of Punjab, and founded the school of internal medicine. He instructed his students to write a book each and thus came into being Agnivesha Samhita, the Bheda Samhita, and the Harita Samhita etc. Of these, the Agnivesha Samhita was judged by the doctors of the time to be the best, most authentic and most complete text of internal medicine. All the original copies have been lost, but Charaka retrieved this book from an original. The other texts written by the disciples of Atreya, except for the much smaller Harita Samhita, have never been found. Lord Atreya's school of internal medicine continues to the present day, and remains the basis of the traditions of the Ayurvedic physicians. The normal length of the student's training appears to have been seven years, followed by a test, but the physician was to continue to learn through his life through texts, direct observation (*pratyaksha*), and inference (*anumana*). In addition, the *vaidyas* attended meetings where knowledge was exchanged. The practitioners also gained knowledge of unusual remedies from lay people who were outside the Ayurvedic community such as hills men, herdsmen, and forest dwellers. The only "sins" recognized in ancient writings are ignorance and ill will.

Ashoka (304-232 BC) was a great patron of Ayurveda and this tradition continued during the succeeding centuries until the reign of Chandragupta Maurya (375-415 CE). A long period of unsettled political conditions, marked by foreign invasions, then followed and Ayurveda faced total neglect. Islamic rulers opposed Ayurvedic practice and the British suppressed it completely. Convinced of their own superior knowledge, Western-style clinics and hospitals were built. Ayurveda barely survived thanks to its native roots and also because the official systems of medicine could not reach in widely scattered and difficult rural areas. The patriotic zeal of the people initiated the revival of Ayurveda as of 1916 CE and over the last 50 years the original **Ashtanga Ayurveda** has developed into following sixteen specialties: *Ayurveda Siddhanta* (Fundamental Principals of Ayurveda), *Ayurveda Samhita* (Classical texts), *Rachna Sharira* (Anatomy), *Kriya Sharira* (Physiology), *Dravya Guna Vigyan* (Materia Medica and Pharmacology), *Ras-shastra* (alchemy), *Bhaishajya Kalpana* (Pharmaceuticals), *Kaumar Bharitya* (Pediatrics), *Prasuti Tantra* (Obstetrics and Gynecology), *Swasth-Vritla* (Social and Preventive Medicine), *Kayachikitsa* (Internal Medicine), *Rog Nidan* (Pathology), *Shalya Tantra* (Surgery), *Shalkya Tantra* (Eye, ear, nose and throat), *Mano-Roga* (Psychiatry), and *Panchka* (Pharmacology).

Today, Ayurvedic hospitals and practitioners are flourishing throughout India and the subject is taught in some fifty universities over a period of five and a half years for the B.A.M.S. (Bachelor of Ayurvedic Medicine and Surgery), with one additional year of internship. Ayurvedic practitioners have been appointed as Honorary Ayurvedic Physician to the President of India. Every year on the occasion of Dhanvantari jayanti, a prestigious Dhanvantari Award is conferred on a famous personality of Medical Sciences including Ayurveda. Kerala promotes research and practices of Ayurveda through well established Ayurveda centers, Ayurveda pharmaceutical companies, and the natural habitat of medicinal herbs and plants on the Western Ghats. The production and marketing of Ayurvedic herbal medicines has dramatically increased along with the scientific documentation of benefits. In last 3 years alone nearly 500 books about Ayurveda have been published in 60 different languages, and programs have been aired by the BBC, Discovery, National Geographic, France 3, etc.

Some milestones in the Development of Ayurveda

- *Rigveda* and *Atharvaveda* 5000 BC.

- *Attreya* and *Dhanwantari* School of Ayurveda 1000 BC.

- *Documented Charaka Samhita* 600 BC, *Sushruta Samhita* 500 BC.

- Muslim Invasions and the Decline of Ayurveda 1100-1800 CE.

- Resurrection of Ayurveda under the Peshwas 1800 CE.

- Ayurvedic medicine taught at the Government Sanskrit College, Calcutta 1827 CE.

- Discontinuation of Ayurveda training by the British 1833 CE.

- Indian National Congress Convention at Nagpur recommends Ayurveda as India's National Health Care System 1920 CE.

- M.K. Gandhi inaugurates Ayurvedic and Unani Tibbia College in Delhi 1921 CE.

- Madan Mohan Malviya establishes Ayurveda College at Banaras Hindu University (BHU), Varanasi 1927 CE.

- Drugs and Cosmetics Act for *Ayurvedic/Siddha/Unani* medicines 1940 CE.

- Chopra Committee recommends fusion of old and modern systems of medicines 1946 CE.

- Pharmaceutical Enquiry Committee under Dr. Bhatia for research in Ayurvedic drugs 1953 CE.

- Dave Committee recommends uniform Ayurveda education 1955 CE.

- Establishment of the Institute of Post-Graduate Training and Research, Gujarat Ayurvedic University, Jamnagar, 1956-57 CE.

- Udupa Committee recommends integrated training in *Siddha and Ayurveda*, 1958 CE.

- Establishment of Post Graduate Institute of Ayurveda at BHU, 1963-64 CE.

- Amendment of Drugs and Cosmetics Act of 1940 for Indian medicines/drugs, 1964 CE.

- Establishment of Central Board of *Siddha* and *Ayurvedic* Education 1964-65 CE.

- Central Council for Research in Indian Medicine and Homoeopathy (CCRIMH) set up in 1969 CE.

- Establishment of Laboratory for Indian medicine, Ghaziabad, U.P, 1970 CE.

- Establishment of National Institute of Ayurveda, Jaipur, Rajasthan 1972-73 CE.

- Publication of Part-I of Ayurvedic *material medica* containing 444 preparations 1976 CE.

- Establishment of Central Council of Research in Ayurveda and Siddha 1978 CE.

- Amended Drugs and Cosmetics Act for import/export of Indian Systems of Medicine 1982 CE.

- Establishment of Indian Medicine Pharmaceutical Corporation Ltd., Almora, 1983 CE.

- Second World Conference on Yoga and Ayurveda, BHU, 1986 CE.

- Jawaharlal Nehru Anusandhan Bhawan founded 1988 CE.

- National Academy of Ayurveda *(Rashtriya Ayurveda Vidyapeeth)* founded 1989 CE.

- Central Scheme for development of agro-techniques for important medicinal plants 1997 CE.

- Implementation of Central Scheme in 32 laboratories for developing pharmacopeia standards of Medicinal Plants/ ISM formulations 1998 CE.

- Establishment of specialty clinic of Ayurveda at Safdarjung Hospital, New Delhi, 1998 CE.

- Information, Education and Communication Scheme for NGOs for propagation and popularization of Ayurveda and other systems, 1998-1999 CE.

- Exhibition of Ayurveda in Mystique India, 1997-1999 CE.

- Vanaspati Van Scheme for large scale cultivation of Medicinal Plants, 1999 CE.

- Ayurveda conference in New York, USA, by PM Atal Bihari Vajpayee, 2000 CE.

- Constitution of Medicinal Plant Board under Indian Systems of Medicine and Homoeopathy, 2000 CE.

- Publication of the 2nd volume of Ayurvedic Pharmacopeia, 2000 CE.

- Constitution of Advisory Group for Research in Ayurveda, 2000 CE.

- Ayurveda mainstreamed in National Population Policy, 2000 CE.

- Publication of 3rd volume of Ayurvedic Pharmacopeia, 2001 CE.

- Publication of English edition of 2nd volume of Ayurvedic Formulary of India, 2001 CE.

- Maiden participation of ISM tableau on Republic Day, 2001 CE.

- Exhibition and presentation of Ayurveda during World Health Assembly, Geneva, 2001 CE.

4.

Ayurveda texts

Ayurvedic remedies in the earlier Vedic literature were written on perishable materials, such as the *taalpatra and bhojapatra,* which could not be readily preserved but stone and copper sheets were used later on. Important hymns dealing with medical knowledge are Rigveda: 7.5, 10.97 and 10.162 while Ayurveda has been called an Upveda of the Atharvaveda which refers to anatomy, physiology, the disease process, and treatments. The important Atharvaveda hymns in this context are: are 1.3, 1.17, 1.22 – 1.25, 2.3, 2.4, 2.8, 2.31, 2.33, 3.7, 3.9, 4.12, 4.13, 5.4, 5.5, 5.22, 5.23, 6.14, 6.20, 6.21, 6.24, 6.25, 6.44, 6.57, 6.83, 6.85, 6.01, 6.95, 6.105, 6.109, 6.111, 6.127, 6.136, 6.137, 7.74, 7.76, 7.116, 8.7, 9.8, 19.34, 19.35, 19.36, 19.38, 19.39. Ritual verses are also to be found in *Rgvidhana* and *Kausika sutra.* Some of these texts refer to the three humors of Ayurveda and also mention *marma, dhamani and sira.*

Internal Diseases

During the Vedic age, a pantheon of demons was responsible for disease that could be cured by medico-religious rites, transferred from the patient to the enemies or undesirable people, dispelled into the ground, or carried away by birds to places where they could no longer be a menace. Early morning (dawn), noon, and early evening (twilight) were considered most auspicious to the healing rituals. While *Atharvaveda* refers to health and diseases in the form of hymns to the healing plant goddesses, *Rigveda* praises male plant divinity. The healing plant **God Kustha** was the remedy par excellence for fever and generally identified with the aromatic costus, exported from Kashmir in the spice trade, and linked with his brother **Soma.** Both Soma and Kustha grew high up in the Himalayas, the birthplace of eagles, the third heaven from earth, and the seat of the gods. Healing plant goddess Arundhati was used in the treatment of fractures and wounds and is identified, among others, with laksa (resinous 'lac'). Thus, Vedic pharmacopeia required a detailed knowledge of the local flora which, along with religious chant by Vedic medical priests, amulets or talismans, were intended to drive out demons and to reestablish equilibrium between man and nature. Later on, Buddhist *sanghas* possessed medical knowledge which facilitated the spread of Buddhism in Bharata and Asia.

The most frequently encountered domestic feminine devil **amiva** in both Rigveda and Atharvaveda, is related to the verb a*mayati* 'to ache' 'to cause pain' from the root *am* 'to seize'. She is associated with malnutrition, hunger and poverty while her opposite a*namiva is* connected with *usha* (dawn), is very auspicious, associated with health, wealth, and longevity. The plant *putrudu* was said to destroy *amiva* as did water and milk products. *Amiva* was also associated with an evil flesh eater responsible for abortions, to be cured with *baja* and *pinga* plants, borne as amulets. Another flesh-eating devil *kanva* could be destroyed by the *prsniparni* plant used as amulets, powder, and headpieces.

Many hymns in Atharvaveda are dedicated to the internal disease demon **yaksma** which afflicts both humans and cattle, is said to enter and possess each and every part of the body leading to the disintegration of limbs, fever, heartache, and pain. In *Taittriya Samhita*, Soma was given thirty three daughters of Prajapati for wives but he took fancy only to Rohini which angered the other thirty two who returned to their father. They were given back when Soma promised to treat them all equally but he again took fancy to Rohini. For breaking his oath, Soma was seized by *yaksma* that could be cured by making an offering to the Aditya, Savitri, Vayu and Agni. The *varana* plant and the *satavra* plant amulets were used to treat *yaksma*, along with gold and guggulu. The scent from guggulu predates its later use as incense and fumigation in India. Closely associated with *yaksma* was the demon **jayanya** who could be driven away by plants, offerings and incantations. The internal disease demon **ksetriya** was variously responsible for leprosy and other skin diseases that could be neutralized by the plant *apamarga* along with barley and sesame. The demon **rapas** attacked the foot and sometimes worked with *yaksma*, leading to eruptions or swelling of ankles and knees. Remedies included water, wind, kustha, cauterization, and barley amulets. It was caused by a worm-like creature from water, possibly *dracunculiasis*, where the worm could be extracted by with barley poultice or amulet. The disease demon **balasa** was responsible for swelling associated with internal diseases that some have equated with tuberculosis. Balasa is said to be the brother of **takman** believed to cause lumps in armpits similar to *vidradha* (abcess) and *visalpaka* (a type of cutaneous swelling). Besides surgery, *cipudru* plant was used to destroy *balasa*, along with amulets.

The most dreaded internal disease demon *takman* was responsible for hot-cold fevers such as malaria. Different types of takman were recognized: daily, every two days, every three days, and every thirty days. In fact, *takman* is put in familiar relationship with *balasa* (swelling), his brother *kasa* (cough), his sister and his evil cousin *paman* (rash). Fever and cough were called Rudra's missiles or arrows and *takman* was likewise believed to strike with a thunderbolt, to possess dreaded missiles, and fiery weapons. The poet healer combined here a magical weather rite with medical charm to ward off *takman* that entered the body like the bad weather. The Frog hymn of Rigveda describes how the cool and wet frog could serve as receptacle for the hot fever; frogs were also used to cure chills in Bohemian Europe. Besides *anjana* (ointment), the divine, aromatic *kushta* plant has been praised as the medicine for all diseases, the choicest among herbs, thrice-born from various divinities, associated with his brother Soma. **Kushta** is said to be borne and acquired by gods from the third heaven, the seat of gods, where immortality made its appearance, where golden boats sail with golden oars, traveling on golden courses to the mountains. His mother's name is ***jivala*** (perennial), and his father's name is ***jivanta*** (life giving) or *uttama* (choicest). He is given three names: **naghamara** (non-destroying), **nagharisa** (harmless), and **kustha** or *uttama* (choicest). Conceivably, the plant was crushed, mixed with fresh butter and rubbed on the patient from head to foot. Its aromatic root was used for cough and fever, as also for fumigation. Associated with *balasa* and *yaksma* are *hrddyota* and *hariman*, or heart burn and jaundice, respectively, both related to ***Agni***, to be treated with water and ointment, respectively, along with charms.

Unlike the internal disease demons like *yaksma* etc, **viskandha** is not said to reside inside the body but causes tetanus from wounds; not much is known about its opposite **samskandha** which is also injurious to the body. *Viskandha* was treated by *anjuna*, a lead amulet, and *jangida* plant which was also effective against *balasa* and *taksman*. Ascites was grouped together with diseases of the abdomen called **udara** that could be treated by laparotomy. Worms or **krimi** were known by a dozen names such as *kururu*, *algandu*, *saluna* etc and ancient healers were able to distinguish their sex and to think of them as living in a society. Various *krimis* were most active during the early rainy season, resided in forests, water, mountains etc, and located in different parts of the body. Treatment ritual consisted of smashing and burning them outside of the body such that a sympathetic action proceeded inside as well. Therapies also included head purgation, vomiting and enema. Jivaka was said to perform the first ever surgery to extirpate worms from inside the head but Atharvaveda tradition dates it much earlier. Germanic tradition, too, mentions worm extirpation, and the two may share a common source, or possibly an import into Germany via trade. **Trepanned skulls** have been unearthed at Timargarha in Pakistan, dated 9th-16th BC, chalcolithic sites of Harappa and Kalibangan in northern Rajasthan, dated 2000 BC, as well as the neolithic site of Burzahom in Kashmir, dated 1800 BC.

External Diseases

Broken bones, fractures and wounds were cured by incantation to the plant goddess **Arundhati** that has close linguistic parallel with German incantations based on the 10th century CE Meresburg spells. The remedy employed was *laksa or lac* derived from auspicious plants believed to possess the same divine characteristics as the goddess Arundhati. Flesh wounds were called *roga*, to be treated with water and herbs. The water called Rudra's urine is said to have come from mountain streams and the sea while plants visanaka, pippali, and munja grass came from the earth. Sand was used to surround the blood vessels and stop blood loss in menstruation and from wounds. Skin disorders were divided into *kilasa* and *palita*, roughly characterized by whiteness and paleness. *Kilasa* was further subdivided into three types and included pustules and leprosy. Besides incantations, preparations from plants like *bhringaraja haridra indravaruni* and *nili* were also used. Hair loss was a bad omen and was to be prevented by the concoction from the plant *nitatn*i along with an elaborate ritual.

Ashtanga Ayurveda

With time, Ayurveda evolved into eight disciplines: *Kayachikitsa Tantra* (Internal medicine), *Shalya Tantra* (surgery), *Shalakya Tantra* (Ophthalmology, Otorhinolaryngology, Ears, eyes, nose, mouth and throat), *Bala chikitsa* or *Kaumarabhritya Tantra* (Pediatrics, conception and pregnancy), *Agada Tantra* (Toxicology including air and water pollution, epidemics), *Vajikarana Tantra* (Sexology), *Rasayana Tantra* (Geriatrics, rejuvenation and longevity), *Bhuta Vidya* (Psychiatry). Shalakya Tantra was led by Videhadhipati Janaka, the King of Videha, near ancient Janakapura in Nepal. Janaka compiled the Videha Tantra which is now lost but some sections have been quoted in Sushruta Samhita. Following Videhadhipati, numerous scholars such as Janaka, Nimi, Kankayana, Gargya, Shataki, Saunaka, and Chakshusya, contributed as well, though the originals are now lost some details are available in Madhava Nidana of the 13th century CE, as also in *Atankadarpana* by Sri Kanthadatta of the 15th century CE. *Kaumarabhritya Tantra* was founded and run by Maricha Kashyapa, the contemporary of Atreya Punarvasu. He lived in Gangadwara in the area of Haridwara and had many disciples, e.g. Vriddha Jivaka, Parvataka, Bandhaka, and Hiranyaksa. The original text of *Vriddha Jivaka*, called Kashyapa Samhita or Vriddha Jivaka Tantra, has been lost but Vatsya in the 5th century CE recovered some details from an original; the tradition survives with the Buddhist physicians of Nepal.

Agada Tantra deals with food poisoning, snake bites, dog bites, insect bites etc. The school of toxicology was founded and run by Kashyapa, also known as Vriddhakashyapa, a contemporary of Atreya Punarvasu who lived in Takshashila. The traditional Toxicology is still practiced by different families of Vishavaidyas (poison doctors) and villagers use them. In ancient times, it was the job of *Vishavaidyas* to protect members of the royal families from being poisoned, as well as to poison enemies of the kings. *Bajikarana Tantra* has no specific text or school of specialists, and is included as a part of Ayurvedic internal medicine in the compendia of Charaka, Sushruta, Vagbhata and others. *Rasayana Tantra* deals with the problems of untimely old age and poor immunity, recorded in the texts of internal medicine.

Shalya Tantra was founded and run by Dhanwantari Divodasa, a contemporary of Atreya Punarvasu, the king of Kashi near Banarasa. His disciples included Sushruta, Aupadhenava, Vaitarana, Aurabhra, Puskalavati, Karavirya and Gopurakshita whose text, except Sushruta Samhita, is lost. Sushruta, son of Kaushika, lived in the area of Koshi River, Nepal. His text is considered to be the best, the most authentic and the most complete book of Ayurvedic surgery. The ancient Ayurvedic knowledge of surgery was well developed at the time of the Rishis and Munis but the medieval healers neither preserved nor developed this tradition. Ayurvedic surgery today is limited only to minor operations such as the lancing of boils, handled by few holistic physicians.

Three traditions of Ayurveda exist today, two of them based on the compendia of Charaka and Sushruta Samhitas, and a third tradition based on Kashyapa. Both the Sushruta and the Charaka Samhitas are the products of several scholars, revised and supplemented over a period of several hundred years. Legends concerning the origins of the text refer to Vagbhata who was the chief physician of king Yudhisthir in *Mahabharata*. The works of Charaka, Sushruta, and Vagbhata are considered canonical and reverentially called the **Vriddha Trayi,** "The Triad of Ancients"; or *Brihat Trayi*, "The Greater Triad". The scholar Vagbhata, who lived in Sindh around 100 BC, wrote a synthesis of earlier Ayurvedic materials in a collection of verses called the **Ashtanga Hridayam** and **Ashtanga Samgraha**. Chakrapani Dutta, a Vaid Brahman of Bengal, wrote books on Ayurveda such as "Chakradutta" and others, and he was also appointed as the Rajabaidya of King Nayapala (1038-1055 CE).

Vangsen, probably in ancient Bengal, wrote a classic Ayurvedic book, simply called **Vangsen.** Later on, a scholar by the name of Madhavacharya composed the book *Madhav Nidan* in the early 8th century CE which is a work on etiology. In the 79 chapters of this book, he lists diseases along with their causes, symptoms, and complications. Fever (*jvara*) was treated in a separate compendium by Madhava (Meulenbeld) but is also mentioned in other compendia. He is thought to have been the prime minister for the Emperor of Vijaynagara and ***Madhav Nidan*** is widely considered the best Ayurvedic book for the diagnosis of some diseases known during that period. After *Madhav Nidan*, the next in line of famous Ayurvedic books, ***Bhav Prakash*** was written during the time that the Portuguese first came to India in 1498 CE by a man named Bhav Mishra of Madras. The period in which he wrote can be pinpointed accurately because in the *Bhav Prakash*, he described the symptoms of a disease called **"Firang-roga"** (Gonorrhoea and Syphilis), which was **introduced to the subcontinent through contact with Europeans** or "Firangi". Bhav Mishra introduced pulse examination and pulse diagnosis. Other works are credited to Sharangdhar, Chakra Dutta, Vaidya Vinod, Vaidya Vamanotsava, Bhaisajya Ratnawali, and Lolimb Raj who wrote the ***Vaidya Jeevan*** in verse form. ***Laghu Trayi*** consists of three works by Madhava, Sarangadhara and Bhave Mishra, published 700 CE, 1226 CE and 1558 CE, respectively. Sarngadhara's Compendium was composed around 1300 CE, consisting of thirty two chapters comprising 2600 verses, and mentions the use of opium for the first time for rejuvenation and as an aphrodisiac. He is also relatively liberal with the use of different poisons and metals. Inoculation was described as a scratch to administer medicine and diagnosis was based on pulse and respiration.

About 200 years ago, Pranacharya Shri Sadanand Sharma wrote the ***Rasa Tarangini***, which was the "base book" for modernizing Ayurveda practices. The book describes the use of many chemical substances as medicine and their use such that Ayurvedic practitioners began to process the traditional herbs in sulphate, nitrate, muriate, phosphate and nitromuriate forms. Sarpagandha (Latin: *Rauwolfia serpentina*), Muriate, Sarpagandha Sulphate, Sarpagandha Phosphate, Sarpagandha Nitrate, Sarpagandha nitromuriate and many others were prepared and tested on patients. The *Ras Tarangini* also mentions "Shankhadrav", which was used internally and externally in many disease conditions.

Translations and Transcriptions during the Raj period

Sir William Jones was appointed Supreme Court judge in Calcutta in 1783 CE and founded the Asiatic Society of Bengal the following year. Many Sanskrit texts were then translated into English while Alexander Hamilton became the first teacher of Sanskrit at the *Ecole des Langues*

Orientales Vivantes founded 1795 CE. He taught Sanskrit to Friedrich Schlegel while in 1814 CE Leonard de Chezy was appointed to the first Chair of Sanskrit at the College de France; his student August Wilhelm was appointed the first professor of Sanskrit in Germany in 1818 CE at the University of Bonn. H. H. Wilson was appointed Boden Professor of Sanskrit at Oxford in 1832 CE. In 1816 CE, philology was born out of the work of Franz Bopp who pointed out the similarities in Indo-European languages and the French Asiatic Society was established in 1821 CE, followed by Royal Asiatic Society in London two years later. Translations followed in rapid succession and Eugene Burnouf in France taught to both Rudolf Roth and Max Muller.

Vedic-Buddhist medical texts were brought to light by H. H. Wilson stationed in Calcutta who pointed out a common connection between Indian, Arabic, Greek and Chinese medicines, almost certainly imported via ISC trade (Chapter 1) as these regions had no medical scriptures of their own (Chapter 15). Ronald Emmeric at the University of Hamburg published several articles on Indian medical texts in the 1970s and translated many texts as well. Two French authors, Alexander Lietard and Allan Zebb, published works on the history of Ayurveda that were instrumental in forcing Charles Daremberg to look seriously at the antiquity of Ayurveda but his bias towards Greek medical tradition led him to make misleading statements. The record was partially set straight by Alexis Cordier and Jean Filliozat in France but the latter passed away in 1982 CE. Dominik Wujastyk is compiling and cataloging a collection of Indian manuscripts at the Wellcome Institute for the History of Medicine in London.

Nagarjuna's *Sushruta Samhita*, a sixth century BC text on surgery, is actually the only treatise for two of the eight branches of Ayurveda. The snake is part of Nagarjuna and is usually depicted as a protective canopy. Unfortunately, Sushruta Samhita was translated so badly that at one point it says cut the feet and hands. In Germany, Franciscus Hessler translated Sushruta Samhita into Latin, published in three volumes 1844-1850 CE. A number of articles on Vedic medicine were published by Adalbert Kuhn, J. Virgil Grohmann, and Heinrich Zimmer while Maurice Bloomfield from Johns Hopkins translated many Atharvaveda hymns which appeared as volume 42 of Muller's *Sacred Books of the East*. Julius Jolly came up with *Medicine* in 1901 CE which presents principal medical authors and their texts along with basic principles of Ayurvedic medicine. German ophthalmologist Elbert M Esser translated Sushruta Samhita while F. G. Muller devoted himself to the history of Asian medicine in nearly 130 articles.

Bower manuscripts were purchased in 1890 CE from a senior Buddhist monk named Yasomitra who lived in the rock cut monastery of Kum Tura near the old Silk Road. Hamilton

Bower passed them on to Rudolf Hoernle, principal at the Calcutta Madrasa, who translated them while the originals were later sold by Bower to the Bodleian library in Oxford. It is really a collection of seven treatises: three on Ayurveda, two on divination and two on incantations against snake bite. The contents have much in common with the medical tradition in India but also practiced widely in Central Asia. Ravigupta's *Siddhasana*, translated from Sanskrit into Khotanese, and other anonymous manuscripts in Sanskrit/Khotanese, further show the **diffusion of Ayurveda into Central Asia**, as for example in the book by Pollock.

In India, Sanskrit texts were translated into the Bengali script in the 19th century CE but Gangadhar Ray (1799-1885 CE) fought for the purity of Ayurveda vis-à-vis western medical traditions. Meanwhile, C. Dwarknath synthesized Indian and western medical concepts into three volumes titled *The Fundamental Principles of Ayurveda*, published in 1954 CE. Several English translations of Indian medical texts now appeared e.g. ***The Surgical Instruments of Hindus*** (Calcutta. 1913-1914 CE) by Girindranath Mukhopadhyaya who also came up with the ***History of Indian Medicine*** 1922-1929 CE. Indian Institute for the History of Medicine at the Osmania Medical Colllege in Hyderabad was established through the efforts of Subba Reddy while Pudupeddy Kutumbiah compared Hippocratic and Greek medicine with Vedic medicine. Priyavrat Sharma and V.W. Karambekar endeavored to find the basis of Ayurveda in Atharvaveda in their book ***Ancient Indian Medicine*** in 1962 CE. Journals like Ancient Science of Life, Journal of Ayurveda, and the Indian Journal of History of Medicine have appeared for the specialist.

All of the *samhitas* show a vast amount of scientific research and patient investigation during the period 2000-200 BC. During the Buddhist era, medicinal herbs were planted along the roads, to be used freely by the public. Veterinary science, nursing and alchemy were developed under the guidance of Nagarjuna around 300 BC. Ashoka took every step for the collection and propagation of medical plants, established hospitals for people, and even animals. King Buddhadisa in 341 CE composed a work containing the elements of all medical sciences, ordered hospitals to be built, appointed physicians one for every town and village, reserved twenty villages for the maintenance of these physicians, appointed medical practioners to care for army, horses and elephants, maintained asylums for the blind and maimed, and carried with him surgical instruments to proffer help whenever needed. The most important Singhalese hall for the sick was founded by Parakrama the Great (1164-1189 CE), himself a physician, where a male and female servant were assigned to care for each patient; the King provided all medication, took care of the needs of the physicians, and himself visited the hall every month to inquire about the treatments and methods. He even took care of sick animals and a legend relates that a bird was taken care of and set free after it was healed. **These practices did not appear in Europe until after the second world war** and even then to a limited extent.

Charaka Samhita

Ayurveda compendia like *Charak Samhita* and *Sushruta Samhita* were documented around 1000 years BC when Sanskrit texts were transcribed in local scripts, such as Begali, Malyali etc, after oral transmission over hundreds and perhaps thousands of years via the Gurukul system. Here, the Guru solemnly directed the students to a life of chastity, truth, honesty, cleanliness and vegetarianism. He was to be free of envy, never to carry arms, to work day and night for the relief of his patients, never to desert them, nor to take advantage of them sexually, to withhold treatment from the enemies of the king, wicked people, to respect confidentiality of the patient's household. The student was to strive with all his being to heal the sick and not to betray the patients for his own advantage. He was required to dress modestly, be collected and self-controlled in manners and behavior, measured in speech, and avoid alcohol and drugs. He was to constantly improve his knowledge and technical skill. At the patient's home, he was to be courteous and modest, directing all attention to the patient's welfare. He was not to divulge any knowledge about the patient and his family. If the patient was incurable, he was to keep this to himself if it was likely to harm the patient or others.

The Charaka Samhita begins with a description of a large and well-attended medical conference of veteran Rishis and Munis (sages), held under the chairmanship of Bharadwaja, to share medical knowledge, and to compile the medical knowledge which had been passed down orally from generation to generation. This stream of Ayurvedic medical knowledge was considered eternal, because it was known by them to have been there since the beginning of time. This historic conference, estimated to have lasted about three years, was a milestone in the history of medicine. After long and complex discussions and debates, several committees were formed to compile full texts about the different subjects of Ayurveda.

Charaka represents the **Atreya school of physicians** and the name Charaka is mentioned in *Samyuktaratnapitakasutra*, a Chinese text of the late fifth century CE, translated from Sanskrit by two Chinese monks Ki-kia-ye and T'an-iao of the Wei dynasty (386-584 CE); Charaka is also mentioned in Bower manuscripts. Here, King Devaputra Kansihka had three intimate friends

Asvaghoas Bodhisattva, his prime minister Mathara, and a famous physician Charaka. The date of Kanishka is also a vexed question but scholars place him 1st–2nd CE. In the Compendium, dated 3rd–2nd BC, the name Charaka occurs as a sort of editor at the end of each chapter while the work is cast as a teaching from the sage Atreya to his pupil Agnivesa whose history is lost in legend. It consists of 120 chapters divided into eight parts: *Sutra-sthanam* (pharmacology), *Nidana-sthanam* (semiology of eight main diseases), *Vimana-sthanam* (general pathology), *Sharira-sthanam* (anatomy), *Indriya-sthanam* (diagnosis and prognosis), *Cikitsa-sthanam* (therapy), *Kalpa-sthanam* (pharmacy), and *Siddhi-sthanam* (general therapy), but each of these large divisions covers a lot more than just the caricatures. The work shows that the author(s) was familiar with the diet of many foreign people: Asians, Persians, Chinese, Greeks and Scythians. It describes 341 recipes from plants, 177 medications from animal products, 64 medications using minerals and metals. It includes diagnosis, treatment, obstetrics, baths, diet, hygiene, education by dissection, amputation, abdominal caesarian, cataracts, sterilization by fumigation, internal anatomy, physiology, etiology, prognosis, pathology, treatment and medicine. Charak's description of human anatomy is actually being studied at London University.

In the Golden Age nothing bad ever happened as the earth and other elements were in harmony and full of good qualities but righteousness waned by one fourth during the Silver Age. Disease arose because good judgment was violated resulting in mental defects such as envy, grief, fear, anger, pride and hatred. All of these had to be suppressed and a good company was to be sought, along with a good life style to calm the senses, be mindful, and be aware of time, place and person. **Natural urges** such as sneezing, farting, coughing, urination, ejaculation, defecation, yawning, clearing the throat, were **not to be suppressed**. Urges for hunger, thirst, tears, sleep, panting due to exertion were also not to be suppressed because suppression of urges was traced to malaise in the corresponding organs. To be suppressed were urges which could cause harm to another person such as rape, robbery or injury. Disease prevention was recommended by thorough catharsis with the aid of enema, *nasya*, massage, and sweating three times a year, at the beginning of rainy season, spring and autumn. **Gymnastics was to be practiced in moderation** as it led to lightness, the power to work hard, firmness, ability to bear discomfort, diminution of humors, and increase in digestion. Excessive exercise was believed to cause tiredness, depletion, thirst, blood-bile, breathlessness, cough, fever and vomiting. Disease could also arise from the contact with contaminated objects, while rats, mosquitoes, earthquakes and bad weather were related to epidemics due to corrupt time, corrupt water and corrupt locale, as a result of unrighteousness or bad actions previously performed. Corrupt rulers could also cause epidemics such as war.

Life ambitions were listed as: **this life, riches, and the next world**. Life span was not predetermined but subject to life style and untimely death resulted from abuse. Heredity was foreseen as familiarity with inherited organ deficiencies. Both the mother and the father contributed to the formation of the embryo to be nourished by nutritive juices. The self of the embryo is the inner self and that is what they call life; eternal, free from disease, old age and death, indivisible and undecaying, uncuttable, unshakeable. Birth is merely a change to a different state. Bad habits were to be given up one at a time and good ones adopted one at a time as well. Humors were to be balanced by regime of contrary quality.

Diseases were divided into those which could be cured (*sadhya*), those that could not be cured but improved (*yapya*) and incurable (*asadhya*). Eight sets of three mention three sources of disease: overuse, underuse and abuse of sense objects, actions or time. The three paths of disease entry are extremities (blood, skin), lethal points and bone junctions (bladder, heart, head etc), and the trunk. Diseases related to the extremities include goiter, spots, diabetes, scrofula, polyps, moles, freckles, pallid skin. Diseases of the middle path include paralysis, seizures, spasms, phthisis, consumption, pain in the joints, anal prolapse, disease of the head, heart and bladder etc. Diseases related to the trunk are fever, diarrhea, vomiting, flatulence, coughing, wheezing, hiccups, constipation, abdominal swelling, rashes, inflammation, abdominal lumps, piles and abscesses. Eight sets of three mentions three types of physicians: imposters, sponsored and accomplished, three kinds of medicine depending upon the sacred, reasoning and good character; three kinds of therapy: internal cleansing, external cleansing and application of knife.

Charaka gave detailed instruction as to the construction of hospital building, staff, supplies, diet, cleanliness, and esthetics. Supplies included ghee, oil, fat, marrow, honey, salt, water, fermented liquors, molasses, spirits, curd, milk, rice, urine, meat and much more. The description depicts a society of abundance. Curds were to be avoided at night and always taken with ghee, sugar, mung bean broth, honey or emblic. Ashoka perhaps had planted the idea of social responsibility in India as his decrees had assured water wells and herbs for the care of animals and people in all parts of his empire. Mukhopadhyaya has documented that *arogyashalas* were the pious acts of first order in pre-modern South Asia. Veterinary medicine was also highly developed for the treatment of horses and elephants in refuges for aged animals.

Sushruta Samhita

The text is presented here as the teachings of Dhanvantari to his pupil Sushruta who is mentioned by the grammarian Katyayana 250 BC as 'a statement by Sushruta'. The final work is divided into six large sections: **Sutra** (origin and divisions of medicine, medical training, therapy, diet, surgery); **Nidana** (symptoms, pathology, prognosis); **Sharira** (philosophy, embryology, anatomy); **Chikitsa** (therapy); **Kalpa** (poisons); and **Uttata** (ophthalmology, dentistry). Sushruta *Samhita* consists of six books arranged into 184 chapters and mentions 1,120 different pathological conditions, including 76 eye conditions, 51 of which were to be treated surgically. The compendium also describes some 650 drugs, 1,120 illnesses, 700 healing plants, 57 animal preparations and 64 mineral concoctions, surgical instruments and procedures. Caustic substances and resin were used to prevent bleeding while bones were enumerated during animal sacrifice, as per *Brahmana* literature of the first millennium BC.

A whole section is devoted to **poisons and antidotes.** Poisons were divided into stationary and mobile, while the former dwells in ten places, the latter had 16 locations; altogether fifty five stationary poisons were described. Slow-acting poisons were treated by the invincible ghee made out of more than twenty five different plants. The Great Fragrance Antidote was to be used to combat poison as also the diet: ghee, curd, milk, honey, cold water, the meat of peacocks, mongoose, lizards, chital, deer, blackbuck and soup made out of them. The most remarkable of these is the **Venomous Virgin** who is a character from the Sanskrit drama and who **became a well known motif in medieval European medical and religious lore**, appearing in the literature of France, Germany, England, Spain and many other countries. This tradition first appeared in Europe in the *Secretum Secreteroum*, a Latin translation of the Arabic *Kitab Sirr al-Asrar* (possibly from a Syrian source). Vagabhata explains that a venomous virgin is a girl who has been **exposed to poison from birth** and thus has become poison herself. Dalhana quotes from some earlier source:*If she touches you, her sweat can kill. If you make love to her, your penis will drop off like a ripe fruit from its stalk.*

Kashyapa Compendium

Only one fragmentary Sanskrit manuscript covers *Kashyapa's Compendium*, just as *Bhela's Compendium* and Vagabhata's *The Tome of Medicine* are available only in fragments. The first manuscript in *Kashyapa's Compendium* was discovered by Haraprasad Shastri in Kathmandu in

1898 CE, consisting of only 38 palm leaves whose copies are to be found in Bibliotheque Nationale in Paris. The second manuscript of the text came into the hands of Hemaraja Sarman sometime before 1938 CE, consisting of palm leaves numbered 29-264. A short text called *Kashyaparsiproktastricikitsatasutrya* has been discovered in a Chinese translation by Dharmadeva who went to China in 973 CE and died there1001 CE. It details principally the diseases of women and children, and their treatment. Prajapati asks the goddess Revati, **Lady Opulence**, to fight on the god's side so she turns into a disease figure called Jataharini and enters the womb to take away what has been conceived. She also figures in Sushruta's Compendium as one of the nine *grahas*. Three kinds of child snatcher are described; curable, improvable and incurable; divine, human or animal. Cures included a Rohini bath and magic known as She-Elephant which had the same value as the Great Horse Sacrifice.

Vagbhata Treatise

Ashtanga-Samgraha forms the last and the most recent volume of the three main books. Compiled by Vagabhata, born in Sindh around 100-200 BC, it found its way to **Tibet** and thence to **China and Japan**. It is therefore clear that medical traditions in these countries owe much to Ayurveda. He was taught medicine by his father Simhagupta, and he could have possibly been the great-grandson of the famous medical author Ravigupta who lived around 600 CE. There is no doubt that **Vagbhata's** *Heart of Medicine* towers above all others and represents the greatest synthesis of Vedic medicine. A second major work ascribed to Vagbhata is known as *The Tome of Medicine* but its relationship with the *Heart of Medicine* has remained a scholarly debate. The work emphasizes daily and seasonal regimes along with six savors that could be combined into 63 possibilities, according to the mathematical principles of Lilavati by Bhaskara, and Paninian grammar; **medical and mathematical traditions converge** here as nowhere else.

5.

Globalization of Ayurveda

Before the dawn of history, an extensive chalcolithic culture connected lower Indus valley with the plains of Mesopotamia and Asia Minor (Turkey). The presence of cylinder seals and "Persian Gulf" type seals in Mohenjo-Daro, Channu-Daro, Lothal, and elsewhere in the ISC sites, indicates that these cities were in contact with Sumeria and Babylon by sea trade. *"The Aegean world into which Greeks penetrated…had already absorbed many cultural elements of West Asiatic origin"* (West cited from McEvilley). During the 3rd - 4th millenium BC, the ISC goods reached Mesopotamia and Dilmun trade (Failaka, Bahrain and Oman) was established by 2400 BC (Chapter 1). Around 1500-1300 BC, the Silk Road linked Bharat, China and Bactria (Afghanistan) to the Near East and the Mediterranean while Phoenicians bought gold, silver, ivory, apes and peacocks from "Ophir" (Bharata). Indus Script and Egyptian hieroglyphs may date back to 3200 BC and may form "the earliest system of writing in the world". Evidently, the colonizers from the Indus valley took urbanization, medicine, mathematics and writing to Mesopotamia, rather than the other way around. Wheeler concedes:

> *"In each of three lands so accessible to one another the immensely complex idea of an evolved civilization (or a writing system) should, within the narrow space of some five or six centuries, have emerged spontaneously and without cross-reference, is too absurd to merit argument".*

The obelisk of Shalmaneser III (cf 860 BC) shows imported Bharata elephants and the palace of Nebuchadnezzar depicts logs of Bharata teak. During the Orientalizing period around 700 BC, Greek mercenaries, artists, and poets brought Babylonian astronomy and mathematics to Greece. Direct **Greek-Bharata contacts** occurred in the Persian empire of Cyrus which was erected on the ruins of the Assyrian empire in the **sixth century BC** that included the Royal Road from Sardes to Nineveh. In 515 BC, Darius extended Persian control to the Indus, creating a new satrapy of Hindush and settled Bharata mercenaries in the empire; a colony of Vedic Hindus was located in the Sumerian city of Nippur and Persepolis documents frequently mention Bharata. Actual names and dates assure of Bharata presence at Persian courts during the pre-Socratic period where Greeks were also present, and Ctesias reports Bharata elephants in Babylon during 500-400 BC. During Achaemenid period, Kharosthi alphabet, in the northwest Bharat, was of Aramic origin and Mauryan art shows Persian influence; so contact with the West undoubtedly existed before Alexander.

Civilizing the whole world, ***krinvantum vishvamaryam,*** had been a declared mission of the Vedic Hindus from the time immemorial. The unimpeded contact between Vedic-Buddhist Bharata and Greece through Persia lasted at least until 490 BC. The work of Pythagoras, Heraclitus, Empedocles, Parmenides and other pre-Socratic philosophy falls during this era; Vedic physiology and Ayurveda had diffused into Greece by the time of Plato. The early periods of philosophy in Greece and Bharata contained many shared elements: the problem of the One and the Many, the Cosmic Person, Monism, and many others. Heraclitus actually purveyed an Upanisadic doctrine in considerable detail so transmission from Bharata is clear, possibly via Persia. Pythagoras visited Bharata and established a retreat along Vedic lines in Greece. Assuming the earliest Upanishads around 500-800 BC, diffusion from Bharat into Greece appears logical, not the other way around. The vast network of Bharata-Greek contacts via both land and sea routes resulted in much cultural exchange over hundreds of years and Astronomy reached Greece as well; Gargi-samhita described the **origin of astronomy**:

> *"The Yavanas are barbarianss yet the science of astronomy originated with them and for that they must be reverenced like gods".*

In Asclepius one finds the infiltration of the eastern tradition into archaic Greece. Wandering seers from Vratyas, Jains and Ajivika traditions had found all the way to Greece via Persia. Browzing (cattle imitation) was a common ascetic vow in Vedic tradition that was also practiced in Mesopotamia. Diogenian cynicism involves Shaivite practitioners migrating from India to Black sea, while the edicts of Ashoka mention seers, embassies, medical and religious missions to his contemporary kings in the West. Pre-Islamic Iran had been transmitting Vedic knowledge to Egypt for over two millennia and to Greece for over one millennium. Bharata soldiers formed part of the Persian army under Xerxes (468-465 BC) and again under Darius III which fought Alexander at the historical Gaugemela battle in 331 BC. Bharata supplied Persia with chariots, horses, steel swords to fight against the Greek tribes who then united against Persia and gave rise to Greece as a nation.

All **ancient and medieval western medicine until the 17th century CE was based upon the theory of humors of Ayurveda.** Pre-Christian healing rites of the Druids, Greeks, Celts,

Germans and Slavs had something in common with Ayurveda as well. Apollonius of Tyana came to Bharata from Greece and took back much of the knowledge with him. During the Middle Ages and the Renaissance, the spice trade brought many Ayurvedic herbs to Europe. The **alchemical traditions from Europe to China were based on Ayurveda** during this same period as **alchemy was heavily proscribed by the Church** in Europe. Hildegard of Binger (12th CE Germany) used many Ayurvedic herbs like the long pepper (pippali), gems and minerals. Ficino mentions many Ayurvedic herbs (Triphala, aloe, saffron, cinnamon and cloves) and formulae in his work: *The Book of Life*.

The healing art of Ayurveda had spread outside of the strictly Vedic community around the 6th century BC. People from China, Tibet, the Greeks, Romans, Egyptians, Persians and many more came to learn about this world medicine and the religious scriptures it sprang from. Ayurveda all but established Islamic medicine and helped lay the foundation of modern European medicine. People who criticized and rejected Vedic ideation copied freely from it and passed it off as their own accomplishment. The fallacy of medical and scientific thinking, particularly in Greece and Rome, is detailed in Chapter 16. Under Charaka and Sushruta ca. 1000 BC, **bone setting, cataract extirpation, plastic surgery, casesarian and rhinoplasty reached a level not known to Europe until the 18th century CE.** The EIC learnt many of these in India and exported the techniques to Europe who then despised India for the lack of surgical tradition.

6.

Ayurveda Instruction

Ayurveda was taught at two major centers of learning in ancient Bharata: **Takshshila (Taxila) and Nalanda**. Legend has it that Taksha, an ancient king who ruled in a kingdom called Taksha Khanda (Tashkent), founded the city of Takshashila ("belonging to the King Taksha"). Taksha was the son of Bharata and Mandavi from the epic Ramayana, while in Mahabharata the Kuru heir Parikshit was enthroned at Takshshila where the epic was first recited by Vaishampayana, a disciple of Veda Vyasa, at the behest of the seer Vyasa himself on the occasion of Janamejaya's (Parikshit's son) 12 year-long *Sarpa-Satra Yajna* (Snake Sacrifice). Takshshila was a Vedic/Hindu and Buddhist center of learning from the 6th-7th century BC to the 5th century CE, and formed the **very first university in the world**. Panini, Jivaka, Bhiksu, Vyadi, Nagarjuna, Chanakya, Brahmadatta and Junaha were associated with Takshshila and written accounts of it were composed by Plinus, Strabo and historians who accompanied Alexander. Generally, a student entered Takshashila at the age of sixteen to study the Vedas and the Eighteen Arts, which included skills such as archery, hunting, and elephant lore, in addition to the law school, medical school, and the school of military science.

Ayurvedic practice was flourishing during the time of Buddha (around 520 BC), and some of the important physicians of this period include Nagarjuna, Surananda, Nagbodhi, Yashodhana, Nityanatha, Govinda, Anantdev, Vagbhatta etc. who ushered in the Golden Period of Ayurveda. During the reign of Ashoka, Takshshila became a great Buddhist centre of learning and it is believed that the Mahayana sect of Buddhism took shape there as well. The last Maurya emperor, Brhadratha, was assassinated 185 BC and Takshshila was **ruled by Bactrian Greeks** 183-90 BC when the Indo-Scythian chief Maues overthrew the last of Greeks. Around 25 CE Gondophares, founder of the **Indo-Parthian Kingdom**, conquered Takshshila. An inscription dated 76 CE reads: *'Great King, King of Kings, Son of God, the Kushana'* (maharaja rajadhiraja devaputra Kushana). The **Hephthalites** swept over Gandhara and Punjab 460–470 CE, leading to the wholesale **destruction of Buddhist monasteries** and stupas, and Takshshila never recovered.

Takshshila lay at the crossroads of three major trade routes: the royal highway from Pataliputra; the north-western route through Bactria, Kapisa, and Peshawar; and the route from Kashmir and Central Asia, via Srinagar, Mansehra, and the Haripur valley, across the Khunjerab pass to the Silk Road. Takshshila ruins are situated about 32 km (20 miles) north-west of Islamabad Capital Territory and Rawalpindi in Punjab, just off the Grand Trunk Road, 549 meters (1,800 ft) above the sea-level. In 1980 CE, Takshshila was declared a UNESCO World Heritage Site. The main ruins are divided into three major cities, each belonging to a distinct time period. The oldest of these is the Bhir Mound, dated sixth century BC; the second located at Sirkap was built by Greco-Bactrian kings in the second century BC; finally the third and last city of Takshshila is situated at Sirsukh and relates to the Kushan kings. A number of ruins of Buddhist monasteries and stupas also belong to Takshshila e.g. stupa at Dharmarajika, the monastery at Jaulian, and the monastery at Mohra Muradu. The city is mentioned by the Chinese monk Fa-Hsien, who came to Takshashila in 405 CE while Hieun Tsang, another Chinese monk, visited Takshashila in 630 CE. Fa-Hsien noted free hospitals run by donations from pious citizens and recorded the **first ever organized, cosmopolitan, institutionally based, medical care and civic hospital system anywhere in the world**:

> *"The cities and towns of this country are the greatest of all in the Middle Kingdom. The inhabitants are rich and prosperous, and vie with one another in the practice of benevolence and righteousness…The heads of Vaishya families in them establish in the cities houses for dispensing charity and medicine. All the poor and destitute in the country, orphans, widowers, and childless men, maimed people and cripples, and all who are diseased, go to these houses, and are provided with every kind of help, and doctors examine their disease. They get the food and medicines which their cases require, and are made to feel at ease; and when they are better, they go away of themselves".*

Nalanda in Sanskrit means *giver of knowledge*, (possibly from *nalam*, lotus, a symbol of knowledge and *da*, to give). According to the Kevatta Sutta, in Buddha's time Nalanda was already an influential and prosperous town, thickly populated, though not yet a center of learning. Sariputta, the right hand disciple of the Buddha, was born and died at Nalanda and Buddha himself stayed there several times in Pavarika's mango grove. According to one sect of Jainism, Mahavira was born in the village of Kundalpur in the Nalanda region and is believed to have attained Moksha at Pavapuri, also near Nalanda. Some parts of Nalanda University were constructed by Ashoka e.g. the Sariputta Stupa, and Nagarjuna is said to have taught there. The main University was however established under the patronage of the Gupta emperors, notably Kumaragupta, and flourished between 427 CE and 1197 CE, thanks to the patronage of Buddhist Emperors like Harshavardhana and Pala kings. According to Tibetan sources, five great Mahaviharas stood out: Vikramashila, the premier university of the era; Nalanda, past its prime but still illustrious, Somapura, and Jaggadala, all under a coordinated state supervision. The Tang Dynasty

Chinese pilgrim Xuanzang left detailed accounts of the university in the 7th CE, how the regularly laid-out towers, forest of pavilions, dharmikas and temples seemed to *"soar above the mists in the sky"* so that from their cells the monks *"might witness the birth of the winds and clouds"*. Xuanzang states:

> *"An azure pool winds around the monasteries, adorned with the full-blown cups of the blue lotus; the dazzling red flowers of the lovely kanaka hang here and there, and outside groves of mango trees offer the inhabitants their dense and protective shade…The lives of all these virtuous men were naturally governed by habits of the most solemn and strictest kind. Thus in the seven hundred years of the monastery's existence no man has ever contravened the rules of the discipline. The king showers it with the signs of his respect and veneration and has assigned the revenue from a hundred cities to pay for the maintenance of the religious."*

Nalanda University was built with red bricks entirely, marked by a lofty wall and one gate, eight separate compounds, ten temples, meditation hall, classrooms, lakes and parks. The library was located in several, nine storied, buildings known as *Dharma Gunj* (Mountain of Truth) or *Dharmaganja* (Treasury of Truth), *Ratnasagara* (Sea of Jewels), *Ratnodadhi* (Ocean of Jewels), and *Ratnaranjaka* (Delighter of Jewels) and housed hundreds of thousands of volumes. Nalanda covered 1 sq km, eight large halls some six stories high, 300 lecture halls, 1500 professors, 10,000 students; clothes, meals, housing were free, subscribed by the king and the well to do. It attracted pupils and scholars from Korea, Japan, China, Tibet, Indonesia, Persia and Turkey and remained the greatest center of learning from 427 to 1197 CE. A vast amount of Tibetan Buddhism, both the sutric Mahayana and Vajrayana traditions, stems from Nalanda teachers and traditions. Mahayana Buddhism, followed in Vietnam, China, Korea and Japan, was born within the walls of Nalanda while Theravada Buddhism was also taught at Nalanda but to a lesser extent. The Buddhist scholar Dharmakirti (ca. 7th century CE), one of the founders of philosophical logic, as well as one of the primary theorists of Buddhist atomism, taught at Nalanda.

In 1193 CE, the Nalanda University was **sacked by Bakhtiyar Khalji**, a Turk. The Persian historian Minhaj-i-Siraj, in his chronicle the *Tabaquat-I-Nasiri*, reported that thousands of monks were burned alive and thousands beheaded as Khilji tried his best to uproot Buddhism and plant Islam by the sword; the burning of the library continued for several months and *"smoke from the burning manuscripts hung for days like a dark pall over the low hills"*. The last ruler of Nalanda, Shakyashribhadra, fled to Tibet in 1204 CE at the invitation of the Tibetan translator Tropu Lotsawa (*Khro-phu Lo-tsa-ba Byams-pa dpal*) who visited the site in 1235 CE to find it damaged and looted; a 90-year-old teacher, Rahula Shribhadra, still instructed a class of about 70 students but an incursion by Turkish soldiers caused them all to flee. The destruction of the temples, monasteries, centers of learning at Nalanda and northern Bharata are responsible for the demise of ancient Vedic-Hindu-Buddhist scientific thought in mathematics, astronomy, alchemy, and anatomy, etc as well as with the decline of Buddhism.

The site of Nalanda is located in the state of Bihar, about 55 miles south east of Patna. The ruins of Nalanda University cover an area of 14 hectares over an area of about 150,000 square meters near the Surya Mandir, a Hindu temple, but almost 90% of it remains unexcavated. The Nalanda Museum contains a number of manuscripts, and shows many of the excavated items while a multimedia show, installed on 26 January 2008, recreates the history of Nalanda in a 3D film narrated by Shekhar Suman. Four more sections in the Multimedia Museum include: Geographical Perspective, Historical Perspective, Hall of Nalanda, and Revival of Nalanda.

A consortium led by Singapore and including China, India, Japan and other nations will attempt to raise one billion USD to revive Nalanda University near the ancient site (*New York Times* December 9, 2006). Nalanda would largely be a post-graduate research university containing: School of Buddhist studies, Philosophy, and Comparative Religion; School of historical studies; School of International Relations and Peace; School of Business Management and Development; School of Languages and Literature; and, School of Ecology and Environmental Studies (*The Times of India* May 11, 2008). The objective would be "*aimed at advancing the concept of an Asian community...and rediscovering old relationships.*" Yet, this laudable goal falls far short of the need to revive enthusiasm in the Vedic-Buddhist past as the people responsible for such undertakings are themselves not sensitive to it.

University Curriculum

The subjects taught at Nalanda covered every field of learning, Buddhist and Hindu, sacred and secular, foreign and native. The students studied science, astronomy, medicine, logic, metaphysics, philosophy, Samkhya, Yoga-shastra, Vedas, Buddhism as well as foreign philosophy. The *Katha, Mundaka, Svetasvatara, Prasana, Maitreyo, Mandukya, Brihardaranyaka and Chandogya Upanishads* deal with physiology, psychology, philosophy, embryology, anatomy and mention two great anatomists Yajnavalkya and Aitareya. Anatomical knowledge was derived not only from the ritual sacrifice of the horse, which called for the recitation of name of each part of the body as it was cut, as per specific hymns of Rigveda but also from human cadavers submerged in cold water for several days for gradual decomposition of the soft tissues; the organs thus revealed were correlated with the surrounding structures. Vedic gods are generally believed to be the personifications of the natural forces. However, *Brihadaranyak* Upanishad mentions that **Rig, Yajus and Sama** were all produced by the God of death, i.e. **from the study of the dead bodies**. In contrast, dissection of the human body was permitted in the Western tradition only in the last few centuries. Yet, several white reductionists have **created anti-history** by writing that dissection was a European tradition.

Vedic sacrifices were meant to regulate and modify the functioning of the bodily universe so as to realize the powers of God who had created the external Universe. The contradictions and confusions in the interpretation of Vedic hymns may stem from the attempt to ascribe them to natural phenomenon whereas in reality the universe of the Vedic seers had no exact replica outside their own bodies. The gods coupled themselves with a wife of their own creation, namely **Speech**, and metaphorized the knowledge as manifestations of the external forces to explain the locations and workings of the human body. Sushruta mentions that all **Gods** described in the Vedas have a **permanent existence in the body**. Rele concludes: *"Vedas are books on the **physiology of the nervous system** written by different Vedic seers"*. In fact, *hatha yoga* has been described as a means to control the autonomic nervous system and Gita as a psychological treatise aimed at unifying the mental powers which could not have been written without a detailed knowledge of the functioning of the nervous system.

The **Vedic anatomy** listed 500 of the 513 muscles, 360 bones, 800 ligaments, 300 veins, 500 muscles, 7 layers of skin, in the human body along with sutures, lymphatics, nerves plexus, adipose tissue, vascular tissue etc. The anatomy and **physiology** of the nervous system were known in detail to the Vedic seers who named different brain structures from the resemblance with the corresponding parts in animals (horse, bull, cow, dog, sow). The various parts of the nervous system are personified as gods, animals, rivers, oceans, seas, strands, poles and the functions they perform, albeit in the language of natural phenomena in the habitat of the Rishis. Human central nervous system is divided into the right and left hemispheres (heaven), separated from the spinal cord (earth) by a cleft, so described as Rodasi in the book addressed to Vishvedevas.

In the Vedic pantheon, the god **Tvastri** remains obscure; he created Agni, fashioned the thunderbolts for Indra, shaped the whole world with his axe, but he was at last overpowered by his own creation, as his son Vivasvat was killed by Indra, and thereafter he took shelter in the harem of the gods. Tvastri could well be the ectoderm whose gradual multiplication and organization are separated during development by a groove into the upper (heaven) and lower (earth) portions, as if hatched into two. The four ventricles are the abode of the gods: **Thalamus is Agni, Cerebellum is Pushan, Pons is Rudra, Corpus Striatum (caudate and putamen along with many other deep elements inside the hemispheres) is Surya, Indra is the ceberal cortex, Manu is the spinal cord**. The morphological appearance of these regions in the adult matches well the physical attributes assigned to these gods in Vedic hymns while the physiological role of these sub organs of the brain is compatible with the actions ascribed to these gods. Furthermore, the birth of the gods follows the embryological differentiation during development (Figure 3 adapted from Rele).

Ribhus are the three sets of fibers through which the gods transmit their desires, while the **thunderbolts** are the **afferent and the efferent fibers** that connect the spinal cord with the brain. The efferent fibers later radiate into the whole cortical area of the brain as **Corona Radiata**, which carries almost all neural traffic to and from the cerebral cortex and forms **Savitri** in his concrete form. The **Maruts** have been associated with storm and wind, fathered by the braided hair Rudra (Pons) and the mother oceans (**Ventricular fluid**), who helped Indra to overcome Vitra. They are said to have kindled fire, make the earth wet with ghee, milk and honey, carry on their activity with unabated vigor, all of which could mean the elaboration of glandular secretions in the periphery, responding to central nerve impulses or the Maruts. **Parjanya** is generally considered a subordinate deity though nothing in the world could exist without him as he is all pervading and stimulated by Mitra Varuna and the Maruts, all of which is compatible with reflex activity.

The hymns to the **Ushas** are the most beautiful of the Vedic verses, daughter of the sky, sister of night; she generates Surya and Agni by riding the chariots (vagus nerve) to the nerve centers in medulla oblongata. The three **strides of Vishnu** are the three relays of afferent impulses from the spinal cord (earth) to the brain (heaven) via medulla oblongata. **Aditi** is both the daughter and mother of **Daksha**, compatible with the center of conscious motor activity (Rolandic area) in the cerebral cortex, one half inch on either side of Sulcus of Sylvius. **Adityas** are the sons of Aditi and could well be the seven conscious motor centers in the Rolandic area of the brain. **Brihaspati**, as controller of speech, lies immediately below the Rolandic area and represents both the conscious and subconscious activities of the mind i.e. thought and speech or Indra and Agni, as described in the hymns. **Soma** is mentioned as a plant that drops from heaven to the earth; this suggests the flow of the **ventricular fluid** from the brain to the medulla oblongata in the form of cerebro-spinal fluid that surrounds the brain, stimulates the voice, awakens thoughts, and gen-

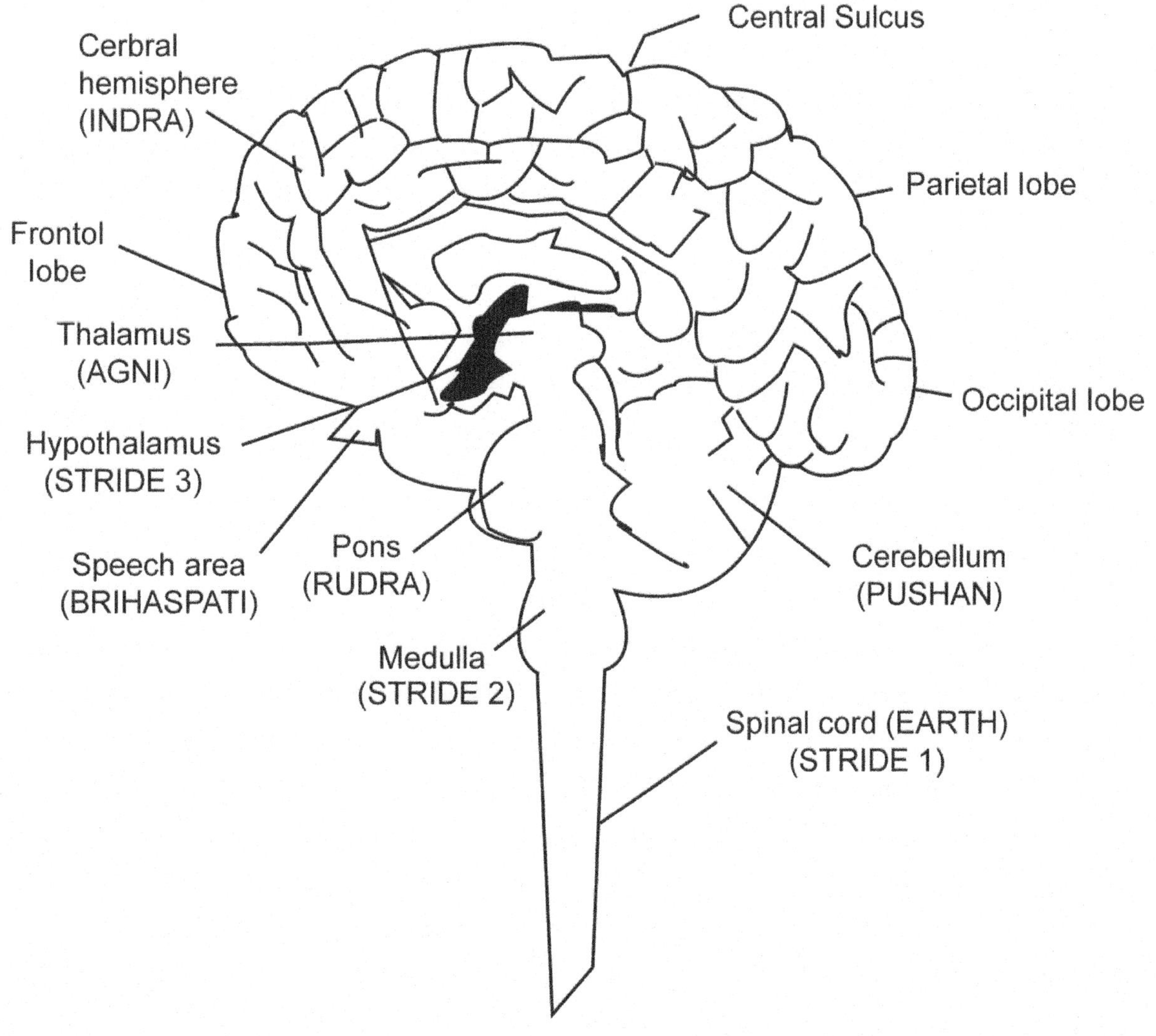

Figure 3. Symbolic Metaphors in the Vedas Related to the Brain.

erates efferent impulses from the brain. The activity of corpus striatum and the thalamus, metaphorized as Surya and Agni, respectively, is coordinated by the cerebro-spinal fluid personified as **Varuna** who towers far above all deities of the Vedic pantheon, and who flows as rain through heaven (brain) over the terrestrial regions (spinal cord) to permeate the soil (muscles, tissues etc); Mitra works with Varuna without the knowledge of Indra.

The **seven rivers of the ISC** region could well be metaphors for the seven tributaries of Sarasvati (cerebro-spinal fluid) that open into **seven** openings of the **sense organs** (two each in the ears, eyes, nose and one of the mouth). The water that flows in these seven rivers is the nerve impulse due to the pressure in the ventricular cavities commanded by Soma. The seven lovely floods by which Indra covered the oceans are the **surging desires** generated by the seven sensory openings which Varuna, lord of the ocean, liberates by his occult power of Maya. Indra is said to have cast his thunderbolt over ninety floods, meaning the efferent connections between the cerebral cortex and the spinal nerves. The ninety racing steeds, together with the four which Vishnu sets in motion, are the impulses from the spinal cord (Vishnu) moving along these nerves.

Embryology was a subject of considerable speculation in *Aitarey, Taittiriya and Kaustaki Upanishads*, and mothers received advice regarding prenatal influences. The cosmological knowledge in the Vedas could really be embryology, composed in a language to suit the grandeur of the all pervading macrocosm. The constitution of the individual was decided by the sperm, ovum, season, food, and gunas, at the time of fertilization. This is to be contrasted with the passive role assigned to the female in Greco-Roman and Christian traditions (chapter 15). *Hiranyagarbha*, the golden egg, the originator of all beings that existed even before the first breath of gods, the only god among all gods, is no other than the producer of the species to which it belongs i.e. a fertilized ovum. The sensory activity of the infant is very dull for three days after birth but afferent impulses are perceived by the tenth day of the extra uterine life. **Ashvins** are described as performing a host of functions in various legends in a large number of Vedic hymns. The legend of Saptavadhari has remained a riddle but could be understood as the rescue of Atri from the fourth ventricle by Ashvins immediately preceding the birth, and for many days thereafter, such that efferent and afferent activities are finally reconciled.

During a symposium on stem cell research, sponsored by All India Biotech Association, Dr. Matapurkar remarked: The epic *Mahabharata* (3000 BC) describes Gandhari as a mother of 100 sons called Kauravas, the eldest of them being Duryodhana:

"No woman can give birth to 100 children in her lifetime, that too all males and of the same age... (Kauravas) were products of a technology that modern science has not even developed yet",

They were created by splitting a single embryo into 100 parts, each of which was grown in a separate *kund* or container, as per a verse in Mahabharata under the chapter *Adiparva*.

"In other words, they not only knew about test-tube babies and embryo splitting but also had the technology to grow human fetuses outside the body of a woman-something that is not known to modern science," (PTI, MAY 04, 2002).

Ayurveda considers that the proper care of children is the foundation of a culture. An ancient Vedic verse states: *"The One God has entered into the mind, born at first, he plays within the child"* (cited in Frawley) and is worshipped in Bharata as Krishna. **Pediatrics** was an integral part of Ayurveda instruction for the well being of the child by oil massage, appropriate nutrition, herbal support, as well as spiritual imprinting through myths and legends. Various texts describe the entry of semen, fertilization, even the thoughts and emotions of the fetus and the manner in which they are influenced by those of the mother and her diet. Acharya Sushruta has clearly defined hereditary diseases in Su. Sh. 24/6 as stemming from vitiation of sperm and ovum but other Rishis had their own explanations: Acharya Charaka described it as *Kulaja Roga*, Acharya Bhela described it as *Prakritibhava*, Acharya Vagabhata described it as *Kulajaj* and *Kulodbhava*, and Acharya Yagyavalkya described it as *Sanchari*. Geriatrics was also a part of Ayurveda to be treated with rasayans, gems, tonifying herbs, pranayama and yoga.

In texts dating back to 1000 BC, **breath** was the prime mover in physiology along with the bile and the pituitary gland. It was known that heart received impure blood, sent it to the liver, and received pure blood, in contrast to the Greco-Roman traditions (Chapter 16). **Urine analysis** was well developed and **pulse** diagnosis was exceptional; Pythagoras later learnt it from India and imported it into Greece. **Nosology** was also highly advanced and diseases were classified according to symptoms, the organs involved and anatomical situation. Kashi (Benares) specialized in surgery while many places in South Bharata taught alchemy and toxicology. **Vaccination** was described in Dahnvantari's *Sacteya* and came to be known in Europe only in the 18th century CE. Sushruta lists 760 medicinal plants many of which have now entered the western materia medica. Life force in plants was scientifically demonstrated by J. C. Bose (1850-1937 CE).

Hypnotism originated in India as well, although the words 'hypnosis' and 'hypnotism' both derive from the term "neuro-hypnotism" (nervous sleep), coined by the Scottish physician and surgeon James Braid, as explained in his major book *Neuropnology* (1843 CE). Braid based his practice on the work of Franz Anton Mesmer and his followers that gave rise to "Mesmerism" or "animal magnetism". Braid discusses hypnotism's historical precursors in a series of articles entitled *Magic, Mesmerism, Hypnotism, etc., Historically & Physiologically Considered,* where he draws analogies between his hypnotism and ancient spiritual practices such as Hindu yoga and meditation as well as the *Dabistan-i Mazahib,* or the "School of Religions", an ancient Persian text. Chinese texts record that this practice was brought in from India and even **reached England in 1700 CE.** Modern applications of hypnosis include: pain management, weight loss, alleviation of skin disease, anxiolytic action after surgery, psychotherapy, habit control, general relaxation, and improved stamina for sports.

7.

Conceptual and Philosophical Background

Western understanding of the universe is based essentially on an objective analysis of the material body and its relationship to the physical world around it. When one considers psychology and the mind/body problem, the question is asked 'is this really scientific'? In the West, the body is believed to give rise to the mind. In contrast, the holistic view of ancient sages, seers, and rishis, postulates that each level of being grows out of the one above it; out of the mind arises the necessity for a physical existence. Western dichotomy stems from the Greek Atomists who saw matter as chunks of inert atoms moved by an external energy. This gave rise to the dualism between spirit and matter, mind and body. At the beginning of the 20th century, the atom was no longer considered hard and solid but mainly empty space filled with subatomic particles. This view too was discarded in the 1920s in favor of the Quantum Theory of a continuous dance of energy particles that saw everything as different manifestations of the same reality. The great metaphor of Shiva Nataraja, lord of the cosmic dance, beautifully portrays this kinetic universe in which all things, from the majestic movement of the great galaxies down to the persistent agitation of sub-atomic particles, are in a state of flux.

Modern medicine places exaggerated emphasis on somatic and physiological processes because science has become an objective approach to the subjective world. People who use conventional medicine usually do not seek treatment until they become ill; there is little emphasis on preventive treatment. The main causes of illness are considered to be pathogens like the bacteria or viruses, or biochemical imbalances, to be dealt with drugs, surgery, radiation, and the like. Whereas Allopathy, defines health as the absence of disease, a definition based on a negative, the World Health Organization (WHO) posits that it is a state of complete physical, mental, and social well-being. It views health as a balance of physical, mental, emotional, and spiritual wellness whose disruption stresses the body and can lead to sickness, much like the holistic tradition of Ayurveda.

The Vedic seers followed an approach diametrically opposite to that of modern science. They turned within and fathomed all the levels of their inner life to finding a common source of existence. If they could fathom the ultimate source of their own "Self" they would find the origin of all things in nature. Rishis transcended pure consciousness to connect with the cosmic intelligence which was the source of all the laws of nature and they called it Veda. This could only be approached by stepping outside the rational thought process by meditation. The **Creation hymn** from the world's most ancient living scripture Rigveda, excels in the abstract ideation by seeking the origin in a primary principle, not related to a deity, *logos* or unmoved mover.

1. *Then there was not non-existent nor existent: there was no realm of air, no sky beyond it.*

   What covered it, and where? And what gave shelter? Was water there, unfathomed depth of water?

2. *Death was not then, nor was there aught immortal: no sign was there, the day's and night's divider.*

   That one thing, breathless, breathed by its own nature: apart from it was nothing whatsoever.

3. *Darkness there was: at first concealed in darkness, this all was indiscriminate chaos.*

   All that existed then was void and formless: By the great power of warmth was born that unit.

4. *Thereafter rose desire in the beginning. Desire the primal seed and germ of spirit.*

   Sages who searched with their hearts' thought discovered the existent's kinship with the non-existent.

5. *Transversely was their severing line extended: what was above it then, and what below it?*

   There were begetters, there were mighty forces, free action here and energy up yonder.

6. *Who verily knows and who can here declare it, whence it was born and whence comes this creation?*

   The gods are later than this world's production. Who knows then whence it first came into being?

7. *He, the first origin of this creation, whether he formed it all or did not form it,*

   Whose eye controls this world in highest heaven, he verily knows it, or perhaps he knows not.

In other hymns, Time is seen as Creator whereas in still others Sacrifice is the creator. It is indeed astounding that modern developments in science, particularly cosmology, seem to echo some of the insights of these great seers and sages, almost like emanations from the Big Bang. The seers of the Vedas and Upanishads had gained two astounding insights although these have emerged in modern science only very recently. The first is the concept of ***Anantakoti Brahmanda*** billions of galaxies or universe. The second is the concept of vast eons of times through which creation passes, the single day of Brahma being of 4.32 million years with a night of equal duration, so that a year of Brahma closely approximates the age of planet Earth. Perhaps this knowledge came to the Vedic seers in an enhanced state of consciousness which forms the prime principle of creation. Thus, we are simply creations, or manifestations, of a cosmic consciousness, much like the expansion following the Big Bang. Whereas sensory experience is real for the western mind, for the yogi, all is in the mind only.

While the Vedic seers also fashioned path-breaking technology in such diverse fields as agriculture, architecture, animal husbandry, metallurgy, chemistry, astronomy, medicine and mathematics, the most creative minds sought the source of consciousness itself, and built up the science of Yoga and Ayurveda, based entirely upon introspection. The yoga-sutras of Patanjali give us a seminal textbook for exploring the deeper recesses of our being that were taken up in the West only with C.G. Jung and the post-Jungian Transpersonal Psychology. Albert Einstein's famous remark that *"science without religion is lame, religion without science is blind"*, makes a very important point. Before him, the Cartesian-Newtonian-Marxist paradigm of thought had postulated an unbreachable dichotomy between matter and spirit. Einsteinian revolution, Heisenberg's Uncertainty Principle, Quantum mechanics and extra-galactic cosmology, are beginning to discern the outlines of a convergence between science and spirituality.

Yoga posits that the mind and body relate to each other by an intermediate level of existence, called ***prana***, which takes the shape of the physical body of the host. Kirlian photography has shown that after amputation, or after plucking of a leaf, the energy pattern of the whole persists for a while. The material body is only the secondary sheath which is constantly changing by the manner in which prana acts upon it. If breath is ignored, breathing will be controlled by the centers of the brain but when one becomes aware of the breathing process, we can gain control over subtle processes of the subconscious. The human body, consisting of 50-100 million cells when healthy, is in harmony, self-perpetuating and self-correcting, just as the universe is. Charaka remarked:

> *"Man is the epitome of the universe. Within man, there is as much diversity as in the world outside. Similarly, the outside world is as diverse as human beings themselves."*

In other words, all human beings are a living microcosm of the universe while the universe is a living macrocosm of the human beings. Everything in this vast universe (macrocosm) also appears in the internal environment of the human body (microcosm). *Jiva atma* in the individual is a reflection of *parama atma* or the universal soul. Each soul's inherent preferences lead it to make choices consistent with its *dharma*. Within 24-48 hours of death, an individual loses all predilections, likes and dislikes, because the soul begins to withdraw from the body.

Natural medicine follows a holistic approach and views disease as an imbalance between the mind and body which is ultimately expressed at the physical, emotional, and mental levels of a person. Although allopathy does recognize that many physical symptoms have mental components (for example, emotional stress might promote an ulcer or chronic headaches), its approach is generally to suppress the symptoms, both physical and psychological. By contrast, the natural medicine envisions the symptoms as a sign or reflection of a deeper instability within the person. It therefore tries to restore the physical and mental harmony which will then alleviate the outward symptoms of disease. Holistic medicine is based on the tenet that the human body is superbly equipped to resist disease and heal injuries. However, when disease does take hold, or an injury is inflicted, holistic approach will try to strengthen the natural resistance and healing principles to combat the disease. Results are not expected to occur overnight, but neither will they exacerbate dangerous side effects.

Ayurveda is the Science of Life where we are all part and parcel of nature and health is maintained by using those inherent principles that bring the individual back into equilibrium with its true self. All disease arises first in the mind that is ultimately responsible for maintaining the harmony between *jiva* and *parama atma*. Since an unhealthy body cannot go on the path of yoga, Ayurveda seeks to attain a perfect equilibrium between health, material means, and spiritual goal. Our birthright is to experience the full potential that comes when living harmoniously with our universal nature. While Ayurveda holds that **normality is subjective** and must be evaluated individually, Western logical deduction equates **normality with the numerically majority**. Just as the animals and plants live in harmony with nature and utilize the Laws of Nature to create health and balance within, so also humans should adhere to these very same principles. In essence, Ayurveda has been in existence since the beginning of time because we have always been governed by the nature's laws. Through the extraordinary powers of contemplation, the rishis came up with knowledge that got to be classified into six philosophical systems: *nyaya* (logic), *vaisheshika* (atoms), *samkhya* (causality), *yoga* (body and spirit), *mimasa* (moral behavior), and *Vedanta* (esoteric knowledge), all of which are part of Ayurveda. Though Ayurveda is based on *Smakhya*, it also uses some elements of the *Nyaya and Vaisheshika*.

The Samkhya Philosophy

Attributed to the rishi Kapila, Samkhya envisions **Purusha** (male) and **Prakriti** (female) elements that combine under the influence of the cosmic intelligence called **mahad or buddhi**.

Purusha is the Brahman of the Vedic thought or the Universal soul, as also the principle of *prakriti*, but has no qualities or gunas (**sattva, rajas, and tamas**) which exist in perfect balance before the union. The whole Vedanta can be summarized thus: **"Man is God, I am God, I am everywhere"**. Brahman or the Universal soul is described thus in *Mundaka Upanishad* of the Vedic period:

"That which cannot be seen, nor seized, which has no origin, which has no properties, which has neither ears nor eyes, which has neither hands nor feet, which is eternal, diversely manifested, all pervading, extremely subtle and imperishable, the wise regard it as source of all beings and creation".

Brahman of the Eternal Energy is also described in human form in *Rigveda*:

"A thousand eyes are the heads of a man-cosmos, a thousand his eyes and thousand his feet ! He is all that is, all that was, all that will be...From his mind, originated the moon, from his eyes, the sun, from his mouth the fire, and from his prana, the air came forth. From his navel originated the space, and from his head the heaven; the earth originated from his feet, and directions came from his ears".

In *Kena Upanishad* the same idea is expressed in different words:

"That which speech cannot express but through which speech is expressed...That which thought cannot conceive but through which thought is thought...That which sight cannot see but through which sight sees...That which hearing cannot hear but through which hearing is heard...That which breath cannot breathe through which breathing is breathed...That, indeed is the immensity and what is here worshipped".

During the later epic period, *Gita* portrays Brahman thus:

"Supreme Eternal Brahman, which can be called neither being nor non-being...without any senses, unattached, supporting everything, free from qualities and enjoying qualities...within all beings, immovable and also movable, by reason of its subtlety, imperceptible, at hand far away is That. Not divided amid beings, it devours and it generates. That, the light of all lights is said to be beyond darkness, wisdom, object of wisdom to be reached, seated in the hearts of all".

The union between purusha and prakriti produced **Ahankara** (ego) and and **Manas** (cosmic mind) which then differentiated into **Tanmaras** (five senses), **Panchamahabhutas** (five elements), **Jnanendriyas** (five sense organs) and **Karmendriyas** (five action organs). From the unmanifested, pure consciousness arose ether under the subtle vibrations of **AUM.** Ether then manifested into air and fire; the latter liquefied some elements to give rise to water which then solidified into earth. Thus, man became the microcosm of nature (macrocosm) and various gods are mere metaphors for different philosophical levels of existence. The trident of Shiva is symbolic of sattva, rajas and tamas, the snake around his neck is time and destruction, the tiger skin on which he sits represents the desire. Rigveda says that the universe was built (not created) by Vishvakarma, venerated by all traders one day after Lakshmi worship on Diwali, as described in *Mahanarayana Upanishad*:

> *"The something in which all things assemble and disperse, on which the gods have their seats, is that, the imperishable, the supreme firmament… That something with which space and heaven and earth are filled, by whose means the sun warms, by whose means the water generates life, is That order and Truth, the supreme Brahman of the sages? Navel of the universe that sustains all"*.

Katha Upanishad describes the relationship between cosmos and the phenomenal worlds thus:

> *"Body is like a chariot, of which soul is the owner, the intellect is the driver, the mind plays the part of reins, senses are the horses, and the world is their arena"*.

Different Branches of Yoga

The various manifestations of nature, metaphorized as gods, have philosophical significance as stepping stones to reach Brahman. The theory of *Karma* was meant to instill righteous conduct througout life which determined rebirth where account had to be settled with so many people, places and situations. Liberation was possible through Yoga which dissolves karma and the microcosm then merges with the macrocosm. **Ahankara** separates us from others due to *adhyaropa* which is illusion from ignorance of the real object. Ahankara controls the three defense systems of the body: aura, skin and immunity, and in excess ahankara allows the entry of toxins and foreign material into the body. Patanjali's **Raja yoga** starts with **hatha yoga** to discipline the body and mind, and it finally **reverses the sequence of samkhya** with its two principles (Purusha and Prakriti). Although Patanjali compiled the *yoga sutras*, in some traditions the original teacher of yoga was named *Hiranyagarbha* (cosmic mind or Brahman); Manu emanates from him and all yogis trace their lineage to this cosmic mind. **Gayatri** mantra was revealed to Vishvamitra for intuitive wisdom and to expiate all *karma*. Although intellect is required for self-realization, intuition finally transcends intellect for the final union with God. After negation of all qualities by **neti neti**, only God remains as **tat tvam asi**.

Gita is **Karma yoga** where selfless work is a prelude to **Bhakti yoga** for total surrender to one's divinity for reunion with God. Karma Yoga is contained in the Kriya Yoga described by

Patanjali. *Jnana yoga* is the most difficult path as it uses the mind to transcend ignorance and forms the synthesis of various philosophical traditions: *Uttara mimamsa* or advaita by Vyasa which is the basis of Jnana yoga; *Purva Mimamsa* by Jaimini where rituals are used to placate gods; *Samkhya* **creation** by Kapila; Patanjali's *Raja Yoga* where Brahman is untouched by Karma to create the world; *Vaiseshika* of Kanada rishi which is a scientific analysis of causes and events; *Nyaya* of Gautama rishi where Ishvara is responsible for creation. *Maya* or prakriti endows qualities on Brahman who becomes Ishwara, Jesus, and Rama, whereas Buddha's Middle Way is addressed to a single universal reality.

These different types of Yoga have been the subject of much authorship, and practical advice has been provided in the following chapters. In contrast, Tantra Yoga has been largely neglected since the the arrival of the British who destroyed many erotic sculptures, burned most Tantric scriptures and eliminated the Devadasi tradition as Temple prostitution although London was a major hub of sex slavery in the era of Victorian vanity (chapter 1). The patriarchs worshipped male dominance and feared female power which was held responsible for the downfall of man in Genesis. The revival of Tantra in recent years has permitted to appreciate its central importance as follows.

The principles of *tantra* were well established by the 200 BC and envisaged a fusion of the male and female duality by harnessing the sexual energy for awakening higher consciousness; therefore, the seminal fluid was not to be wasted. The Tantric creation follows Samkhya such that Krishna with his consorts are purusha and prakriti (Shiva and Shakti) respectively. Shakti is revered in many forms but primarily as vulva where union with Shiva is accomplished with many mantras and rituals. In the Kali manifestation, Kali is *Shakti*, garland of human heads is the wisdom, her red tongue signifies rajas which impel all activity, the sword and the severed head signify karma. She is the consort of Shiva on whose body she is often standing; Shakti is also depicted as Mahalakshmi and Sarasvati. The revival of Tantras was the work of Nagarjuna, Ashvaghosa and others under the cover of Brahminism, although it had existed much prior to the Vedas, and is depicted in Mohenjo-Daro seals as *Mahayogi*.

The total fusion of the male and female principles was to be achieved by the arousal of the *kundalini* which lies dormant at the base chakra but tantric practice makes it ascend to the crown *chakra* for total union between Shiva and Shakti known as *ardhanaareeshwara*.The division into *Shiva* and *Shakti* makes one aware of the distinction between male and female but their sexual attraction to each other reminds them of their oneness. As Shakti dances, a whole world of images is formed. The human body is represented as an inverted tree where *sahasrara* in the crown center receives energy from the earth, flows through the body, ends at the muladhara, and spreads into space as an aura. The spinal column is compared with the central axis of Mount Meru, encompassing both the female Ida (left) and the male Pingala (right) aspects (see chapter 9). Great care must be taken to assure that the kundalini does not ascend or descend either through the Ida or Pingala but through the sushumna. While other yogic traditions preach asceticism and repression to experience truth, Tantra raises the sexual ecstasy to the highest degree to merge all of the accumulated karma back to the pure energy which leads to enlightenment, thus reversing the genesis. Tantra becomes the most powerful and rapid tool to enlightenment, within a period of six to twelve months. Whereas science looks backward in time, Tantra reverses the common sense by a process termed *paravritti* where psychophysical organism itself contains the origin, and the whole world is seen as revolving around oneself.

Wall sculptures of Khajuraho and Konark depict the technique of transcending sex so spirituality eventually replaces sensuality. Here, one is enveloped into a feeling of peace and sacredness by freeing oneself of sexuality depicted on the outer wall, and then the devotee enters into the presence of all peaceful Shiva inside the temple. The sculptures are created as similes of egolessness and timelessness, as in samadhi; **bhoga leads to yoga**. All ***Yantra*** symbols are representations of the *yoni* (vulva) which generates world and time. All yantras are graphic forms of *mantras* and each *mantra* has its yantra. Shri yantra is so complex that meditation on it reverses genesis and one is forced to come face to face with the act of creation. The whole system including the yoni originates from the seed at the center of the yantra where interwoven triangles represent the creative energies subdivided into specific forces. Rings and outer circles of the lotus petals represent the world reality as it unfolds by the action of Mahakala and Mahakali. One worships either the female genitals (a downward facing triangle), or a lotus flower and a lingam, or one adores the image of the goddess as a beautiful girl. This is sometimes called the Lotus-Stem meditation. The image is washed, worshipped, garlanded and acquires power in time.

In ancient times, specially trained power-holding females, temple dancers, etc initiated the males via specific yogic postures to permit prolonged and better sex and put ejaculation on hold. Both the lingam and yoni were exercised to attain prolonged erection and penetration, without ejaculation. The best time for tantric sex was during menstruation when her "red sexual energy" was at its peak. The white male seed was either ejaculated in the yoni as sacrifice, or prolonged orgasm was restrained and sublimated to drive the energy through the chakras. Osho Rajneesh observed that on an average the coitus lasts for a minute and one wants sex the next day. If coitus can be prolonged to three minutes, one may not want it again for a week while prolongation to seven minutes may extinguish desire for three months; an extension to three hours may free a person for an entire lifetime, leading to samadhi. The Tantrist can learn to have an orgasm through meditation alone or not have one despite intense sensation to the Genitals .This is done by slowing, or even stopping, the breath through pranayama, by focusing attention on the third eye, or by concentrating on a white light. The separation of orgasm from ejaculation does not lead to the loss of energy and vitality. Chanting the mantra **Kling Kling Kamdevya Namaha** for about one hour every day brings about the power to prolong ejaculation for a long time. At the time of ejaculation, it is imagined that the semen is being sacrificed for a holy purpose.

Before the session, protection is generally asked of Elders, Shiva and Shakti, by making a circle of flour or salt around the devotees and speaking out loud that mischievous spirits cannot cross this line. After a while, a particular presence will become the personal guide or *Ishtadevata*. The **ha-tha** count 1-4-2 (inhale-retain-exhale) is used for the purification of the body which can also be accomplished by water, fire and earth. All of these traditions believe in advaita: dissolution of the self into the Absolute: **tat tvam asi**.

Secret tantra ritual may include any or all of the following: a feast (representing food, or sustenance), coitus (representing sexuality and procreation), the charnel grounds (representing death and transition), defecation, urination and vomiting (representing waste, renewal, and fecundity). Many rituals are performed on cremation grounds (real or symbolic) to understand the dissolution of everything. In a ritual termed *chakrapuja*, couples (married or not) indulged in meat, alcohol, fish, particular grains and sexual intercourse. Again, the orgasm was either restrained or the semen collected in one container to be tasted by everyone as *prashad*. The Tantra is directly related to the phases of the moon, just as the farmer plants downward growing crops when the moon is waning and upward growing grain when the moon is waxing. Tantra starts at the new moon cycle and reaches nirvana towards the full moon. Each pair of the eleven-plus days between the new and full moon is assigned to one of the chakras to cure specific disease problems. Yogins arrange their mensrual periods to coincide with the new moon and food, sex, etc are related to the moon cycle. In modern practice, the maithuna ritual is meant to maintain the partners at the brink of orgasm for 32 minutes and as soon as possible after that the orgasm is encouraged (Frost). Also taken into account are the daily routine, the seasons, the week and the month. One *tantric* tradition, also found in European and Japanese sources, was to bring virgins to lie with the sick old king; **virgins were brought to sleep with Gandhi when he was recovering from a fast**. No intercourse is involved here but the exchange of energies was meant to join the male and the female principles.

Buddhist tantra does not recognize Muladhara and kundalini but relies on the mantra: **'Om Mani Padme Hum'** which connects the individual soul to the universal, Mani means jewel, padme is lotus and hum forces the mantra into realization. Jewel in the lotus is the symbolic representation of lingam in the yoni. The energy of mantra is symbolized by a *vajra* and a bell that is constatntly rubbed with a stick to produce a humming sound like the primordial AUM. The conversion of sexual energy into spiritual energy has been described by many authors to include: Swami Satyananda Saraswati, Elizabeth Haich, Sigmund Freud, Barbara Harris Whitfield, and Wilhelm Reich. All of them equate sexual act as human attempt to return to the original, unimpeded flow of cosmic energy. This is symbolized as the great Simurg of Persia carrying a pair of divine lovers, hermaphrodite being in Judaism and Gnosticism, and by an androgynous being in Greek mythology. The Chinese call the cosmic force *Feng Shui* and Tantric temples were built on sites rich in this earth force, such as the top of a hill.

The Panchamahabhutas

Charaka took all elements of Samkhya in reference to the human body, emphasizing the subjective prakriti, and the role of previous karma that determines health at the time of birth. The omnipresent **Panchamahabhutas** combine in an infinite combination of relative proportions such that each form of matter is unique. Constantly changing and interacting with each other, they create a situation of dynamic flux that keeps the world going. In the case of a complex, multi-cellular organism as a human being, **akasha** corresponds to spaces within the body (mouth, nostrils, abdomen etc.); **vayu** denotes the movement (essentially muscular); **agni** controls the functioning of enzymes (intelligence, digestive system, metabolism); **jal** is in all body fluids (as plasma, saliva, digestive juices); and **prithvi** manifests itself in the solid structure of the body (bones, teeth, flesh, hair etc.). Within a simple, single living cell, for example the earth element provides structure to the cell; the water element is present in the cytoplasm and the liquid within the cell membrane; the fire element regulates the metabolic processes, the air element forms the gases therein while the space occupied by the cell denotes akash. Although each element has a range of attributes, only some get expressed in particular situations. The Panchamabhutas flow sequentially from birth to death with age: Akash to Vayu to Agni to Jala to Prithvi; generally, jala and prithvi predominate. Earth dominates between the feet and the knees, water between the knees and the anus, fire between anus and plexus, air between plexus and eyebrows, and ether between the eyebrows and the top of the head, in order of their weight.

Health or sickness depends on the balance between these different constituents that are in perpetual motion in the body, a fact recognized in the West only in the last 100 years or less. The loss of equilibrium can result from dietary indiscrimination, undesirable habits, non-observance of rules of healthy living, seasonal abnormalities, improper exercise, erratic application of sense organs, and incompatibility in actions between the body and mind. The Panchmahabhutas therefore serve as the foundation for all diagnosis and treatment in Ayurveda where the manifestation of disease is taken as a good sign in as much as it reveals a previously hidden aspect of the self to be healed. The following table summarizes the organ-dependent attributes of the five aforementioned elements.

Mahabhuta	Organ	Faculty	Properties	Actions	Taste
Akasha	Ears	Hearing	Sound	Softness, lightness, Porosity	None
Vayu	Skin	Touch	Breath	Dryness, Lightness, Emaciation	Bitter
Agni	Eyes	Sight	heat	Digestion, Maturation	Pungent
Prithvi	Nose	Smell	support	Firmness, Strength	Sweet
Jala	Tongue	Taste	Fat, Fluid	Nutrient, Emollient, Purgative	Astringent

The Three Doshas

Tridoshas, or humors, are formed by the Panchamahabhutas that associate according to their natural affinities. Ether and air combine to form the *Vata dosha* which is located in the colon, thighs, hips, ears, bones and organs of touch. Vata is the driving force for all human activity; it governs movement, transformation, motor and sensory functions, directs nerve impulses, circulation, respiration, elimination, secretions, excretions, fear, emptiness, anxiety, expels toxins from the body, dries out wounds and stimulates healing. Hyperactivity of vata occurs around 4 AM and 4 PM, after the age of 60, after digestion, after food intake that is dry, cold and light, after intense athletic activity, overexertion, intercourse, injury, cold bath, exhaustion, loss of body tissue, grief, anxiety, worry, intense joy, fright, insomnia, loud music, noise and air travel. A vata person has a light body weight, is shy, sensitive, ascetic, and very prone to all *vata* maladies: rheumatism, sciatica, insomnia, nervous disorders, dry skin, constipation, weak bones, infertility, impotence, weak heart, colic, flatulence, varicose veins, etc. Vata is believed to aggravate the duality of pitta and kapha, is not a humoral category in ancient Greek medicine, and is also absent from earlier Vedic literature. Vata becomes irritated by practices such as riding on elephants, horses, camels, cold climate, refrigerated foods, iced drinks, excessive physical exercise. Vata diseases are characterized by pain and include most nervous system disorders, insomnia, tremors, epilepsy, paralysis, arthritis, tissue wasting.

Fire and water combine to form the **Pitta** *dosha* that directs transformation or metabolism of food into nutrients that our bodies can assimilate. Pitta is located in the small intestine, stomach, sweat glands, blood, lymph, and eyes. It produces **dhatus** (body tissue), **malas** (waste products) and doshas (energy) from food. It is responsible for all gastrointestinal secretions, body temperature, hunger, thirst, sight, skin discoloration, intelligence, anger, hate and jealousy. A weakened *pitta* can be healed by food and medication that have a warming effect while products with cooling effect diminish it. Hyperactivity of *pitta* occurs at noon and midnight, in middle age people, during digestion, after hot, spicy, salty or sour food, during fast, prolonged hunger and thirst, hot weather, anger and hate, and intense intellectual activity. A *pitta* person is between vata and kapha, with a well functioning metabolism and urge for physical activity, healthy body, alert, inventive, technical or scientific, good speaker, bald, prone to ulcers, tumors, cancer, psoriasis, inflammation of the lymphatic system, infections, hepatitis, infection of the urinary tract, heartburn, and herpes. Pitta diseases are characterized by fever and burning sensation.

Water and earth combine to form the **Kapha** *dosha* which is located in the chest, throat, head, pancreas, lymph, fat, nose and tongue. It is responsible for lubrication, unctuousness, forgiveness, greed, attachment, accumulation, possessiveness, sexual potency, resistance to illness, patience, inner strength, growth and protection. Cerebrospinal fluid in the brain and spinal column is a type of Kapha found in the body as is the mucosal lining of the stomach. Kapha is hyperactive around 8 AM and 8 PM, after a meal that is oily, fatty, cold, sweet, after excessive water intake, during physical inaction, cold and wet weather, when greedy, miserly and attached to materials possession. A kapha person has a heavy, solid body, overweight, lethargic, secure and self confident. Kapha diseases are characterized by phlegm.

Pitta, Kapha and Vata are like Brahma, Vishnu and Mahesh or creation, maintenance and destruction, respectively that do not exist as structures or materials but play an invisible role as movers and agents of change. They are not separate energies but different aspects of the same energy, present together in an infinite variety of combinations, wherein their qualities overlap and interrelate. Thus, kapha is not mucus but the force that causes mucus to arise. Similarly pitta is not bile but that which causes bile to be produced while vata is not mala but responsible for the formation of waste from food. The three doshas within any person keep changing constantly, due to the dosha qualities of lifestyle, nutrition, environment, time and season. When the doshas are in balance i.e. in a state of equilibrium health is maintained. Charaka explains:

"Vata, pitta and kapha maintain the integrity of the living human organism in their normal state and combine so as to make the man a complete being with his indriyas (sense organs) possessed of strength, good complexion and assured of longevity."

An individual's prakriti is a unique proportion of Vata, Pitta and Kapha while an imbalance between them will cause disease. As the dominant dosha usually has the greatest tendency to increase, one is most susceptible to illnesses associated with that particular dosha. This holistic, individual approach of Ayurveda is **in contrast to allopathy** where everyone is treated in the same manner. Kapha, Pitta and Vata predominate in distinct zones of the body: Kapha predominates from head to diaphragm, including the secretions of nose and eyes and saliva; Pitta predominates in the lower part of the stomach, small intestine to the ileocecal vale, liver, pancreas, gallbladder and spleen; Vata predominates from navel down to include the large intestine, the reproductive organs, legs, and organs of elimination (Figure 4). Whereas the Kapha zone secretions are whitish, those of the Pitta zone are yellow-red and green; Vata zone secretions are brown, purple or black. However, the three *doshas* pervade the entire body though Vata is the most universal of them all. Kapha, Pitta and Vata predominate childhood, post puberty and middle age, respectively, and during winter, summer and autumn, respectively.

Daily cycles of the doshas are: Kapha I 6-10 AM; Pitta I 10 AM - 2PM; Vata I 2 PM-6 PM; Kapha II 6-10 PM; Pita II 10 PM-2 AM; Vata II 2-6 AM. Besides the Vata, Pitta and Kapha dominant bodies, there are seven mixed types: V-P, P-V, V-K, K-V, P-K, K-P and V-P-K (V =vata, P = pitta, K = kapha).

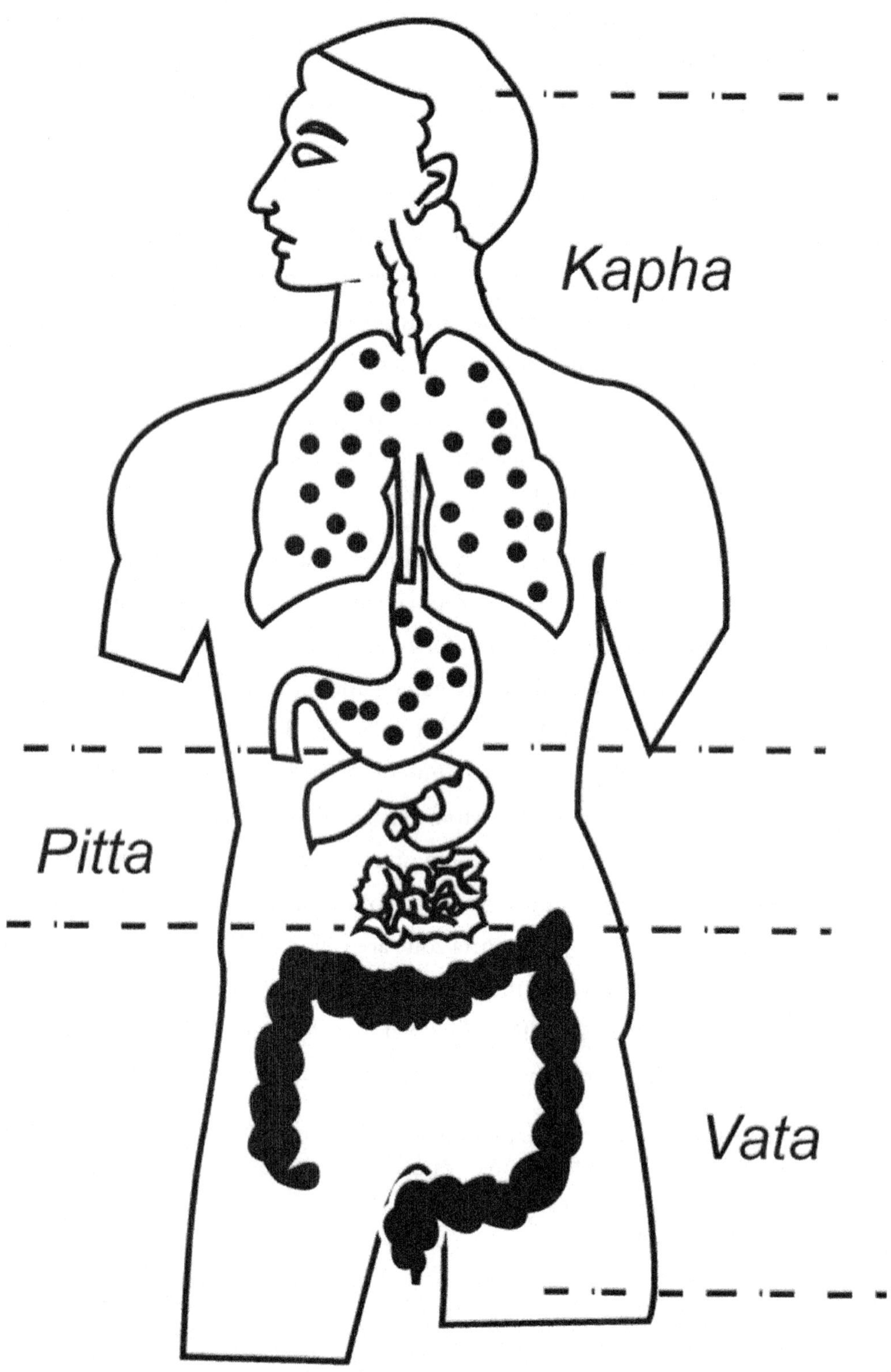

Figure 4. Dosha zones in the human body.

Vagabhata and Charaka have detailed **physical signs of longevity**: prominent forehead; ears small if viewed from front but large when viewed from behind; eyes with distinct white and black parts; thick and well set eyelashes; lips red and protruding; prominent nose with large nostrils; large jaws and mouth; glossy, smooth, white teeth; red, long and thin tongue; big and well formed chin; thin, red, raised nails; large feet and hands, full of flesh and reddish; long fingers; expansive back; spine covered with flesh; deep and resonant voice; glossy and vibrant skin; strong joints covered with muscles and flesh; full of vigor and strength. Body height, measured in finger unit (*anguli*), was to be eighty four times the finger breadth (168 cm or 5'6"). Charaka calculates life span according to forty seven factors.

Each of the three doshas can be subdivided as follows. *Vata* (Vayu) is subdivided into five subtypes. **Prana vayu** moves from the head to the navel via mouth and nostrils to control breathing and swallowing whose dysfunction is expressed as hiccups, bronchitis, asthma, cold, and hoarseness. **Udana vayu** flows in the opposite direction, from the navel to the nostrils and head to control speech and voice whose dysfunction leads to various diseases of eye, ear, nose and throat. **Samana vayu** circulates in a clockwiswe direction around the navel area to control digestion and food assimilation into various tissue; its dysfunction leads to indigestion, diarrhea. **Apana vayu** travels from the navel to the anus and urethra to control elimination of stool, urine, semen, fetal and menstrual blood; its dysfunction leads to diseases of the bladder, anus, testicles, urinary tract, and diabetes. **Vyana vayu** moves from the heart to the periphery and back to the heart in a circadian rhythm to control circulation; its dysfunction results in impaired circulation and fever.

Pitta is also subdivided into five subtypes. **Pachaka** in stomach and small intestines controls digestion whose dysfunction leads to indigestion and anorexia. **Ranjaka** in the liver, spleen and stomach controls blood related activity whose dysfunction leads to anemia, jaundice and hepatitis. **Sadhaka** in the heart controls memory and mental functions whose dysfunction leads to psychic disturbances and cardiac diseases. **Alochaka** in the eyes controls vision and **Bhrajaka** in the skin regulates color and glaze of the skin; dysfunction in these leads to the diseases of the corresponding organs.

The five subtypes of Kapha are: **Kledaka** in the stomach moistens food whose dysfunction can lead to indigestion. **Avalambaka** in the heart regulates energy in limbs whose dysfunction leads to laziness. **Bodhaka** in the tongue controls taste whose dysfunction leads to indigestion. **Tarpaka** in the brain nourishes the sense organs whose dysfunction leads to loss of memory and impairment of function of sense organs. **Shlesshaka** lubrifies the joints and its dysfunction leads to pain in the joints.

Ayurveda generally considers only three types of constitution; in monotypes just one *dosha* predominates, in duo types two have near similar strength, and in the very rarely found third type all three are equally powerful. Each *dosha* thus shares a quality with the other and each has an inherent ability to regulate and balance itself. Most of the physical phenomena ascribed to the nervous system by modern physiology, can be identified with *Vata*, just as the entire chemical process operating in the human body can be attributed to Pitta, including enzymes, hormones and the complete nutritional system. Finally, the activities of the skeletal and the anabolic system, or the entire physical volume of an organism, can be considered as Kapha. Insanity was divided into six kinds due to imbalance in humors. These three humors (Vata, Pitta and Kapha) interact with seven basic tissues or dhatus as well as the three malas (see below) all of which are significantly affected by individual psychological mechanisms as well as by Agni. Yogic asanas exert pressure on the organs to release ama and have been designed to enhance the ability of the doshas to maintain *proper dhatu and mala* functions, as well as the smooth flow of prana in the body.

The Digestive Fire Agni

Agni (fire) is central to the Vedic ideation of the Universe at all levels. On the one hand, it reunites the microcosm with the macrocosm during the elaborate sacrifice rituals around fire and, on the other hand, it constitutes the central process of digestion to transform the panchmahabhutas in the macrocosm to nourish the microcosm. The digestive ability of an individual is directly related to the strength of Agni whose activity varies throughout the day. The maintenance of a good Agni is required for digestion, immune function, resistance to disease, internal secretions, metabolic reactions, cellular transformations, assimilation of sensory perceptions and mental and emotional experiences, vitality, complexion, sight, thermo genesis, the formation of dhatus and of ojas to maintain and repair the body. Agni therefore covers entire sequences of chemical interactions and changes in the body and mind. Agni and pitta are closely connected or even the same and Agni is also subtly related to vata; while both are hot and light, Agni is subtle, dry and acidic. The heat energy to help digestion in pitta is Agni where pitta is the container and Agni the content. Present in every cell, a balanced Agni is vital for health and a disturbed Agni is usually the chief cause of disease.

Ayurveda mentions thirteen types of Agni in the body and mind, according to the conversion and the transformation to be made. The digestive Agni is divided into five types depending upon the action, place, name and ailment. The most important of them is the **_Jatharagni_**, the gastric fire responsible for digestion by the secretion of digestive enzymes and juices in the stomach, duodenum and the small intestines. If the digestive Agni is low, one may experience pain, discomfort, feeling of heaviness or gases gurgling, constipation or loose stools. Jatharagni manifests itself in the body as five subtypes of Pitta: **_Pachak pitta, Rajnak pitta, Alochak pitta, Sadhak pitta and Bhrajak pitta_** located in the small intestines, liver, eyes, brain and skin, respectively. The most important of all is the **_pachak pitta_**, found in the lower stomach and small intestine; when it is strong, the appetite is good. Some authors, such as Joshi, have related specific zones of the colon to particular human diseases (Figure 5).

The **_prapaka_** digestion, under the influence of Jathara Agni, prepares food to be transformed into the dhatus by **_vipaka_** digestion. The influence of jatharaagni first causes the food mass to be converted into a predominantly sweet taste in the kapha zone (stomach), then to a sour taste in the _pitta_ zone (small intestine), and finally to a pungent taste in the vata zone (large intestine); bitter and astringent are digested last. The influence of kapha creates a heavy or sleepy feeling; when food enters the pitta zone, body temperature rises while the vata phase promotes activity. A digestive problem in these zones will exacerbate the respective feelings e.g. increased acidity indicates pitta indigestion. Vata indigestion stems from imbalance in the previous two phases. Jathara Agni exerts its influence on life everywhere e.g. unrefrigerated fruit or milk successively turns sweet, sour and pungent.

Vipaka digestion starts after the nutrients have been absorbed. Dhatus are now formed under the influence of respective dhatu agnis. **_Rasa_** metabolism begins vipaka digestion to produce a substance capable of sustaining the rasa dhatu. But only a portion is taken and the rest is bound by kapha and vata to rakta dhatu in the liver, spleen and the bone marrow. Vata acts as the carrier to take the nutrient to be acted upon by the next dhatu Agni, until all seven dhatus are formed. The end product of vipaka digestion is the **_ojas_** which is causal to immunity and permits every cell to be in direct communication with the nature's limitless intelligence and enlightenment. Agni is increased by pungent, sour and salty tastes, spices like asafetida, ginger, cumin, rock salt, as also by exercise, yoga, pranayama, and staring at a ghee lamp. In contrast to the Western tradition, sweets should be eaten first and salts the last as sweets in the end will stop the digestive process.

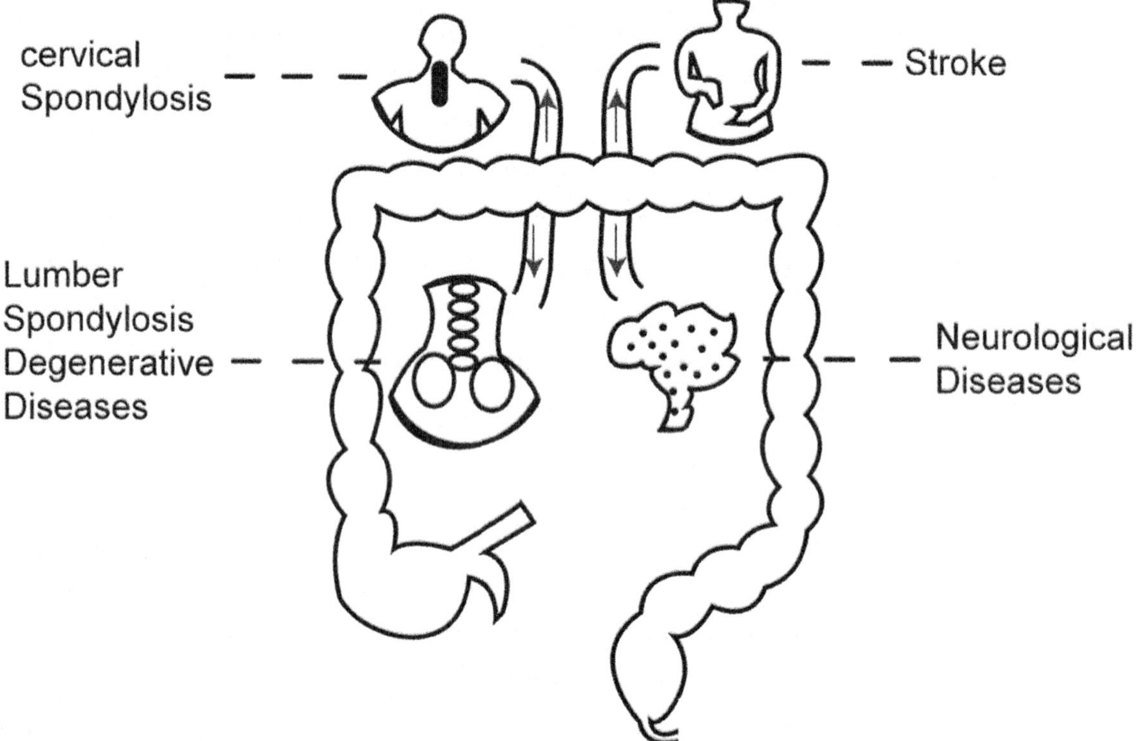

Figure 5. Different zones of the colon related to specific diseases (adapted from Joshi).

The Seven Dhatus

The food cooked by Agni is transformed into seven dhatus under the influence of pitta which form the pillars of the body as well as the mind. *Rasa Dhatu*, derived from the digested food, nourishes each and every tissue and cell of the body and is analogous to the plasma. *Rakta Dhatu* is like the circulating blood; it not only nourishes the body tissues, but also provides physical strength and color. *Masma Dhatu* is equivalent to the muscle tissue for physical strength and support for the *Meda dhatu* or the adipose tissue that also lubricates the body. Meda dhatu forms the support for *Ashti dhatu,* comprising of bone tissues and cartilages whose main function is to give support to the *Majja dhatu* consisting of yellow and red bone marrow tissue that fill up the *ashti* and oleate the body. *Shukra Dhatu* is equivalent to the reproductive tissue for libido, reproduction and stamina. It is said that **3200 successive transformations** are required for the formation of shukra dhatu from the ingested food. As the dhatus support and derive energy from each other, malfunction in one component influences all others. Each tissue has its own Agni which determines metabolic changes specific to it; by products are either used in the body or excreted. As all of the tissues are governed by the three doshas an imbalance in any one of them will desequilibrate the dhatus.

The Ama

Ama is the **undigested food** that remains in the gastrointestinal tract and is the **root of all disease**. Ama accumulates wherever there is a weakness in the body; it is the opposite of Agni. When *ama* becomes too plentiful, it is removed by doshas and transported to the dhatus and debilitates them, leading to a weakened immune system, which depletes or disturbs the digestive *Agni (pachak pitta)* leading to more *ama* or undigested food. The dhatus are no longer formed when all nutrients are gone. The dosha processes that eliminate mala get disturbed which further weakens the dhatus. Ama and mala block the ability of the dhatus to assimilate food and medicine. Ama can remain in the dhatus for years leading to degenerative diseases. Ama can also clog the channels like the intestines, lymphatic system, arteries, veins, capillaries, and genitourinary tract, as also the flow of energy through nadis. An Ayurveda specialist can diagnose the dhatus where ama has accumulated and pinpoint the imbalance in the digestive process responsible for producing *ama*. The symptoms such as coating on the tongue, feeling tired all the time, fecal materials that sinks rather floats, bad breath, abnormal appetite, are all signs of *ama* accumulation. Panchakarma is intended to eliminate ama but it is best to prevent it from forming in the first place by fasting, and herbs Trikat (Triphala, Asafetida, katuk, neem, and aloe). Fasting for one day per week is highly recommended to clean the digestive system. Anti-ama diet includes most vegetables and grains but excludes most fruit, nuts and seeds, dairy products, meats (pork is the worst), oils, alt, sweeteners, cold drinks and tonifying diets.

The Malas

Malas are the various waste products produced during the normal metabolic transformation and the synthesis of the dhatus. If the body is not eliminating malas, it is accumulating *ama* somewhere in the system, thereby necessitating Ayurvedic cleansing to get rid of these toxins. The three primary *malas* are **Purisa** (faeces), **Mutra** (urine) and **Sweda** (sweat). Purisa is the waste remaining after nutrients of digested food have been absorbed in the small intestine; the residue is converted into solid faeces whose consistency depends both on gastrointestinal mobility and the nature of diet. Mutra or urine formation begins in the large intestine where fluids are absorbed into the system. The entire urinary system (kidneys, uterus, bladder and urethra) participates in the formation and elimination of urine to regulate the fluid balance and blood pressure. Any imbalance in urine output may result in kidney stones, urinary infections, cystitis, abdominal pain and bladder disorders. Sweda (sweat) is formed as a waste product during the synthesis of meda dhatu (fatty tissue) and transported to skin pores via the sweda vaha srotas. Sweat controls body temperature and helps to regulate the electrolytic balance. Impaired formation and flow of sweat leads to skin infections, itching and burning sensations over the body, loss of fluid balance, and hypothermia. Ayurveda clearly states that only a balanced condition of doshas, dhatus and malas is **arogya** and their imbalance results in ill health or disease. Pitta and kapha help digestion and vata governs the mobility throughout the process. Any discrepancy or imbalance between these can lead to abdominal heaviness or pain, flatulance, constipation or diarrhea, rheumatoid arthritis, osteoarthritis, low-back pain, asthma, bronchitis as well as stomach ulcers and irritable bowel.

The Six Savors

Six savors or tastes originate from various combinations of panchamahabhutas: earth and water (**sweet**), fire and earth (**sour**), water and fire (**salt**), ether and air (**bitter**), fire and air (**pungent**), air and earth (**astringent**). They **exert heating and cooling effects** to different degrees: pungent is hottest followed by sour and salty; coldest is bitter followed by astringent and sweet. They are also classified as heavy and light: heaviest is sweet followed by salty and astringent while lightest is bitter followed by pungent and sour. They can be either moist or dry: Sweet is the wettest followed by salty and sour, driest is pungent, followed by bitter and astringent. Three tastes increase the trigunas and three decrease them. Vata is increased the most by bitter followed by astringent and pungent; it is decreased the most by salty taste followed by sour and sweet. Pitta is most increased by sour, followed by pungent and salty; it is most decreased by bitter, followed by astringent and sweet. Kapha is increased most by sweet followed by salty and sour; it is most decreased by pungent, followed by bitter and astringent. Sweet is the most nutritive followed by sour, astringent, pungent and bitter. Bitter and astringent are used to treat fevers, infections and traumatic injuries. Sour, salty and sweet are used for long term tonification. Each taste in excess causes damage to the humors but a lack of each taste will aggravate humors. Herbal formulae containing all six tastes are given to children to balance humors, generally 500 mg every morning. One formulation consists of shatavari (sweet), amalaki (sour), rock salt, ginger (pungent), barberry (bitter), and haritaki (astringent).

Sweet, sour and salt destroy wind; bitter, pungent and astringent destroy phlegm; astringent, bitter and sweet destroy choler. Sweet increases blood, fat muscle, bone, nerve tissue, semen, obesity; it causes excess sleep, heaviness, lethargy, loss of appetite, cough, diabetes; it prolongs life, imparts vigor, improves skin voice, hair, decreases Pitta, Vata and toxins. Sour increases thirst sensitiveness, appetite, promotes strength, salivation, helps digestion, increases *pitta*, promotes closure of eyes, dissolves *kapha*, vitiates blood, promotes edema, ulcerations, heartburn and acidity. Salt helps digestion, diminishes *Vata*, increases *Pitta*, causes fainting and heating of the body, aggravates skin diseases, inflammation and blood disorders, causes peptic ulcer, rash pimples and hypertension. Pungent purifies the mouth, stimulates digestion, promotes secretions in the mouth, eyes and nose, reduces edema and obesity, removes excess oiliness, decreases itching, dilates the channels, decreases *kapha* and virility, increases heat, sweating, burning in the throat, stomach and heart, can cause dizziness and unconsciousness. Bitter taste increases roughness, emaciation, dryness, reduces bone marrow and semen, can cause dizziness and eventual unconsciousness, relieves burning, itching, thirst and skin diseases, removes extra water from lymph, sweat, urine, feces, bile and mucus, and aggravates *vata*. Astringent increases dryness of mouth, distension, gas, constipation, speech obstruction, and heart dysfunction; it decreases kapha, increases vata, purifies blood, removes excess water from the body, inhibits excretion of feces, urine, sweat. Altogether, there are **fifty seven combinations** of savors and by choosing the correct one it is possible to balance the three *doshas* in the body.

The Three Gunas

Just as the doshas are the essential components of the body, the three gunas - ***Sattva, Rajas and Tamas*** - are the three essential components or energies of the mind. Ayurveda provides a distinct description of people on the basis of their ***Manasa*** (psychological) Prakriti. Genetically determined, these psychological characteristics are dependent on the relative abundance of the three gunas. While all individuals have mixed amounts of the three, the predominant guna determines an individual's mansa prakriti. In equilibrium, the three *gunas* preserve the mind (and indirectly the body) and maintain it in a healthy state. Any disturbance in this equilibrium results in various types of mental disorders. The knowledge of patient's mind is called **dhi** which is used to increase **dhruti,** the life supporting aspect of rajas, and to elevate **smriti** which causes the patient to stop unhealthy activities. The gunas, like the doshas, can be unbalanced by stress and negative desires such as **kama** (lust), **irshya** (malice), **moha** (delusion and halucination), **lobha** (greed), **chinta** (anxiety), **bhaya** (fear) and **krodha** (anger). Each of these properties is also comprised of sub-types which determine the qualities of that individual.

Sattva, characterized by lightness, purity, compassion, love, consciousness, pleasure and clarity, is pure, free from disease and cannot be disturbed in any way. A sattvic mind has the limitless power of atma while rajas and tamas artificially enhance the functioning of the mind. It activates the senses and is responsible for the perception of knowledge and creativity. **Kapha sattvic** individuals are usually noble and spiritual in character, their nature determined as much by body type as their star constellation. The **Vata sattvic** mind has the ability to make positive changes, to start projects, to have enthusiasm, quick comprehension, good communication skills, flexibility, energy and a strong healing force. **Pitta sattvic** mind makes a good leader who is clear, enlightened, intelligent, warm, friendly and independent. Kapha sattvic mind is calm, stable, loyal, peaceful, compassionate, devoted, nurturing and receptive. **Fruits** are by far the best diet for sattvic people as they **contain large amounts of ether** which controls and balances all other elements. Most vegetables are also good for a sattvic diet but garlic, onion, radish and chilies are rajasic and tamasic. Seeds and nuts, dairy products, ghee, sweet in moderation, most essential oils are good for sattvic people. Sattvic spices include ginger, cinnamon, cardamom, turmeric, fennel and coriander. Sattvic people should avoid meat, fish, eggs, garlic and onions but sometimes can use *rajasic* and *tamasic* spices (cayenne, black pepper, mustard, asafetida and salt) in moderation.

Charaka clearly emphasized the importance of mind in Patanjali's yoga sutras:

> *'The unwholesome action performed by one whose intellect, restraint and memory are deranged is known as intellectual error. It vitiates all the doshas (humors)".*

The sattvic mind is characterized by Charaka as follows:

> *"The persons having dominating sattva are endowed with memory, devotion, are grateful, learned, pure, courageous, skilful, resolute, fighting in battles with prowess, free from anxiety, having well derived and serious intellect and activities and are engaged in virtuous acts".*

Thus, yoga postures without the Ayurvedic discipline, and vice versa, will remain incomplete. Both are required for the total well being due to the interdependence of the body and the mind. Sattva should be cultivated daily through *dinacharya, asanas, pranayama* and meditation (chapters 9, 10, 11).

Rajas is the most active of gunas, characterized by motion, initiative, aggressiveness, and stimulation. All desires, wishes, ambitions and fickle mindedness stem from it. *Vata rajasic* life is indecisive, hyperactive, irritative, anxious, noisy, disruptive, and liable to make superfluous conversations. *Pitta rajasic* mind is often angry, proud, critical, dominating, ambitious, impulsive and manipulative. *Kapha rajasic* mind will manifest attachment, control, greed, material tendency, pursuit of comfort, security and sentimentality. Most spices are rajasic as is pasteurized milk

Tamas is characterized by heaviness, resistance, darkness, dullness, and selfishness. It produces disturbances in perception by the mind, delusion, false knowledge, laziness, apathy, sleep and drowsiness. *Vata tamasic* state is fearful, dishonest, secretive, depressive, self destructive, addictive, pervert and suicidal. *Pitta tamasic* prakriti nurtures hate, vindictiveness, destruction and criminality. *Kapha tamas* is characterized by dullness, lethargy, apathy and insensitivity.

The Subtle Essences

Prana, ojas **and** *tejas* perform vital functions in the body. *Ojas* is the essence of all seven *dhatus* that governs hormonal balance, immunity, intelligence, love peace, creativity and tranquility. It is the "juice" that forms after food has been properly digested and assimilated. When the body is producing ojas, all organs have vitality and receive the nourishment needed by the mind and the body. The whole being hums with good vibrations because the body is imbued with bliss, not pain. However, when the Agni isn't working properly, ojas is is not produced. Ojas is the subtle glue that cements the body, mind and spirit together, integrating them into a functioning individual. Ojas is transformed into an aura through pranayama and such a person is full of spiritual energy and power; he is attractive with lustrous eyes, and a spontaneous and calming smile. Ojas is related to kapha, aggravation of kapha displaces *ojas* and vice versa; the ensuing disorders and can be treated with ghee, milk, ashwagandha, guduchi, meditation and mantras such as AUM. Ojas enters the fetus in the eighth month of pregnancy from the body of the mother. Sex and masturbation deplete *ojas* at the time of orgasm and it is also depleted by anger, hate, worry, sorrow and overwork. Whereas *Para Ojas* exists in a quantity of **eight drops**

within the heart whose loss leads to death, ***Apara Ojas*** is distributed throughout the body. In conditions like HIV, diabetes mellitus, and malnutrition, loss of ojas is a preeminent feature.

Tejas is responsible for the transformation of each dhatu and governs metabolism through enzymes. When tejas is aggravated, it burns away *ojas* and leads to the production of unhealthy tissues such as the tumors, and obstructs the flow of prana. Improper diet, bad living habits and overuse of drugs will imbalance tejas while substances that are hot, sharp, and penetrating directly enhance tejas.

Prana is developed in Sutra 39, Part III, into its five fold dimensions and is causal to life. Prana is the life force responsible for respiration, oxygenation, circulation, motor and sensory functions, an active *Agni*, and works as intelligence in the body. Prana resides in the head and controls mind and memory as well as the heart. *Prana* enters the fetus through the navel to regulate the circulation of *ojas*. Prana gets its nutrition through lungs (air) and colon (food). Thus the lungs and the large intestine are closely connected in Ayurveda as they both replenish *prana*. Longevity requires balanced tejas, ojas and prana as well as a calm mind. Celibacy and spiritual discipline are causal to longevity as are yoga practices.

Indriyas (five senses) act as a bridge between the atma (soul) and manas (mind) on the one hand, and the physical body and environment on the other. Misuse of senses disturbs the equilibrium due to an excess of stimuli, insufficient sensory input, or intake which is morally or emotionally repugnant.

8.

The Disease Process and Management

Charaka observed:

"Perverted, negative and excessive use of sense objects, time and intellect is the three fold cause of both psychic and somatic disorders…Other factors which also cause amadosa are the mental afflictions with psychic emotions such as passion, anger, greed, confusion, envy, bashfulness, grief, conceit, excitement and fear. The self (soul) is devoid of disorders".

The **negative thought patterns** such as anger, criticism, resentment anger, fear, attachment, *ahankar*, repressed emotions, disturb agni and aggravate pitta, vata and kapha, leading to the gradual **loss of *sattva*** due to wrong choices in food and behavior. Criticism indulged over long periods will often lead to arthritis. Anger and worry produce toxins that aggravate pitta, leading to heart ailments, while resentment ultimately engenders tumor and cancer. Guilt always seeks punishment and leads to pain. Excess talking, fear and nervousness dissipate energy and aggravate vata. Possessiveness, attachment and greed enhance *kapha*. Control over thoughts can shape life very positively. Therefore, one should root out all negative thoughts from the mind and concentrate on only the positive ones. Next to worry, hate is just about the worst form of self-destructive mental activity; it poisons the body and mind and its effects are almost permanent. People of kapha constitution are susceptible to kapha diseases that originate in the stomach: tonsilitis, sinusitis, bronchitis, and lung congestion. Pitta constitution is susceptible to diseases that originate in the small intestine: gallbladder, bile and liver diseases, hyperacidity, peptic ulcer, gastritis, inflammation, skin rashes and hives. Vata constitution favors diseases of the large intestine: gas, lower back pain, sciatica, paralysis and neuralgia. Also, if one has no will to live, a long life is not possible. On the other hand, a positive mind definitely favors a long and healthy life. A person who exercises, meditates and thinks positively, is telling his body that he wants to stay healthy. In metaphysical causation, words and thoughts modify the physical self. The way to control life is to control words and thoughts by relaxation, meditation, and concentration, through music and mantras. Brihadaranyaka Upanishada (V.4.5) concludes: *"as is a man's will, so is his action, as is his action, so he becomes"*.

Ayurveda believes that our physical form consisting of mind and senses is preceded by a subtle form, or the soul, which remains unchanged through successive births. At the time of death, some individuals have been documented to experience the sensation of being "out of their body". It is important to maintain the original prakriti or nature in each individual. The aggravation of one or more *doshas* due to smoking, chewing tobacco, breathing in chemical fumes, or eating foods and fruits that have been heavily processed with chemicals causes impurity of the blood which relocates in a region that has weak immunity. One of the main functions of blood is to transport prana which regulates well being. When pranic energy is stagnant or blocked in the meridians or chakras, the prana reaching the cells of the impure region also becomes impure leading to impaired cell function. In Ayurveda, the role of senses is important such that sound, touch, light, taste, odor all affect the disease process. Loud sound and noise can damage health and produce pathological changes in the blood. The second main factor is the misuse of will (**Prajnaparadha)** by perverted actions of the body, mind or speech. Mind is the motor which not only controls our thought processes but also directs respiration, circulation, digestion and elimination. The disease (dis = deprived of and ease = comfort) is believed to proceed in three stages. In **Pragya Apardha,** the intellect becomes identified with our limitations rather than with our unlimited potential. The second stage called **Asatymya-Indriyartha-Samyong,** or the misuse of senses, stems from the preceding loss of *sattva* so the mind loses its ability to make life-supporting decisions, leading to imbalanced *doshas* and the production of ama. In the last stage or **Parinam,** seasons further aggravate the disease. Four kinds of illnesses are: **Nija** (endogenous), **Agantuka** (exogenous), **Manasika** (psychological) and **Svabhavika** (Natural) which can be influenced by climate, hypo- or hyper- activity and malfunction. The disease aggravation is believed to proceed in six stages: **Sancharya** or accumulation with mild symptoms; **Prakopa** or aggravation when *ama* continues to be produced but pulse diagnosis is possible; **Prasara** or migration through *dosha gati* (twice daily migration of doshas) to sites away from its site of origin; **Sthana Samshraya** or augmentation when dhatus are overwhelmed leading to tissue damage and susceptibility to infections; **Vyakta** or symptom manifestation; and **Bheda** or complications due to damaged *shrotas*. Whereas the **Western medicine begins only with stages 5 and 6**, the person has actually been living with the disease since a long time.

Physical Diagnosis: Examination Process

Everything in Ayurveda is validated by observation, inquiry, direct examination and knowledge detailed in the ancient texts. Examination covers the body constitution, pathological state, tissue vitality, physical build, body measurement, adaptability, psychological constitution, capacity for digestion, exercise and age, daily routine, dietary habits, the gravity of clinical conditions, and details of personal, social, economic and environmental situation. The diagnosis involves the eight fold examination (*Pariksha*) as follows.

Prakriti pariksha (face and general appearance). The face is the mirror of the mind and reflects dosha influences. Horizontal wrinkles on the forehead indicate deep seated worries and anxieties. While a vertical line between the eyebrows indicates repressed emotions in the liver, a vertical line on the right side indicates emotions in the spleen. Heavy and puffy eyelids indicate impaired kidneys while a butterfly-like discoloration on the nose or the cheeks means deficiency in iron or folic acid. While vata cheeks are flat and sunken, kapha cheeks are plump. Sharp, blunt and crooked nose indicates pitta, kapha and vata constitution, respectively. Vata, pitta and kapha lips are thin and dry, red, and thick and pale, respectively. Various sections of the lips are related to different organs. Lips should be examined for color, spots, lines, shapes, distortions. Nails are believed to be the waste products of the bones. Vata nails are dry, crooked, rough and break easily; pitta nails are soft, pink, tender and slightly glistening; Kapha nails are thick, strong, soft and very shiny. Each finger and thumb corresponds to an element and an organ of the body. A detailed discussion of self-examination has been provided in the book by V. Lad.

Tissue Vitality (*sara*). The seven vital tissues: lymph (rasa), blood (rakta), muscle (mamsa), adipose (meda), bone (asthi), bone marrow (majja) and reproductive tissue (shukra) are assessed by physical inspection. Lymph in the skin is appreciated by its smoothness, softness, clearness, thinness and the presence of short, deep rooted and delicate hair. The blood content of the body is evaluated from the condition of the eyes, mouth, tongue, lips, nails and soles of the feet. When muscles are in perfect condition, the temples, forehead, nape of the neck, shoulders, belly, arms, chest, joints of the body, jaws and cheeks are covered firmly with the skin. People with healthy adipose tissue have oily skin and healthy hair, nails, voice and teeth. The health of bones is determined by pliable but firm forearms, chin, nails, teeth, ankles, knees and other joints of the body. Healthy bone marrow leads to good complexion and stout, long, round and stable joints. When the semen is perfectly healthy body is strong and cheerful. Additional information is gleaned by assessing: *sambanana* or physical build, ***pramana*** or body measurement in finger breadths, ***satmya*** or adaptibility to change and food options, ***sattva*** or psychic constitution, ***ahara shakti*** *or* digestive capacity to ingest and digest food, ***vyayama shakti*** or capacity for exercise (low, moderate or high), ***vaya*** or age (childhood, middle age, old), prakriti or body constitution (*doshas* and *gunas*), and vikruti or pathological state.

Nadi pariksha (pulse examination). The foremost clinical art in Ayurveda diagnosis, pulse examination can provide deep insight into the history of the disease. Quantum physics has now revealed that the physical nature is essentially vibrational; every organ and tissue in the body has its own vibrational signature. Ayurveda mentions 3.5 million channels in the body that pass through the vital organs. When blood flows from the heart to the periphery and back, it picks up bodily vibrations so a heartbeat can accurately communicate a vast amount of information. The pulse also reveals something about the important meridians that connect the prana waves in the body. The ideal time for pulse examination is early morning on an empty stomach but, in case of emergency, it can be examined at any time of the day or night.

An experienced Ayurveda physician can assess body's nature (prakriti), pathological state (vikruti), imbalances of body type, and even prognosis of disease through the pulse. The physician places his index, middle and ring fingers on the left and the right sides to check vata, pitta and kapha, respectively. The pulse may also be checked at the temporal artery, the carotid artery, the brachial artery, the radial artery, post tibial artery, and the dorsalis pedis artery on top of the foot. By applying different levels of pressure to the artery, an experienced examiner can determine the state of the vital organs. On the right arm, a superficial touch by the index finger is related to the intestine but a firmer or deeper pressure relates to the lung. The middle finger with a superficial touch can detect the status of the gall bladder and that of the liver with a deeper pressure. The ring finger senses the pericardium with a superficial touch and the harmony of VPK with a deeper pressure. On the left arm, the superficial touch reveals small intestine, stomach and bladder, but a deep touch is related to the ear, spleen and kidney, respectively.

Jivha pariksha (tongue examination). Different parts of the tongue are related to different vital organs in the body. A vata aggravated tongue is back-brown, dry, rough and cracked, pitta suffered tongue is red or yellow-green with a burning sensation, and a *kapha* tongue is white coated, wet, slimy. Coatings on the middle part of the tongue indicate toxins in the stomach and small intestine while coating in the posterior portion indicates toxins in the large intestine.

Shabda pariksha (voice examination). Healthy and natural when the doshas are in balance, the voice will become heavy when aggravated by kapha, cracked under pitta, and hoarse and rough when afflicted by vata.

Sparsha pariksha (skin examination). Also used for assessing the state of organs and tissue, palpation is an important clinical method for examination of skin. A vata aggravated skin is course and rough with below normal temperature; a pitta influenced skin has quite high temperature, while with kapha dominance it becomes cold and wet.

Drka pariksha (eye examination). Vata domination makes the eyes sunken, dry and reddish brown in color. On aggravation of pitta, they turn red or yellow and the patient suffers from photophobia as well as burning sensation. High kapha turns the eyes whitish, wet and watery with heaviness in the eyelids. Small eyes that blink frequently show vata predominance. A drooping upper eyelid indicates sense of anxiety, fear, or lack of confidence, all related to deranged vata. Big, beautiful and attractive eyes indicate a kapha constitution. Pitta eyes are lustrous and sensitive to light, with reddened whites and a tendency to be nearsighted. Prominent eyes indicate thyroid dysfunction. The color, shape and size of the iris are related to arthritis, sugar or calcium depletion, deterioration of joints, and sclerosis.

Mutra pariksha (urine examination). A drop of sesame oil *(taila) drop (bindu)* is put in a glass of urine. If the oil disperses the illness is not serious; if it sinks to the bottom then the disease is serious. This test also informs the physician regarding the dosha prakriti of the patient. Ancient texts describe twenty types of diabetes based on specific degeneration of tissues which can be smelled in the urine by an experienced physician.

Mala pariksha (stool examination). If the stool remains floating in water, good health is surmised but if digestion and absorption of food are poor, the stool carries a foul odor and sinks in water. Vata aggravated stool is hard, dry and grey-ash in color while an excess of pitta makes it green.

It is evident from the foregoing that **Ayurvedic examination is sometimes far more detailed than that used in the western diagnosis**. For example, western pulse examination is used almost entirely for heart beats, in contrast to the Ayurvedic method which informs on the state of all of the internal organs. Similarly, the western face examination yields much less information than in Ayurveda which also places much emphasis on skin, tissue, voice, tongue etc all of which are important in the rural setting. Similarly, urine and stool examination in the western medicine are of far more limited scope than in Ayurveda. However, the biochemical analysis in the western medicine has nothing comparable in the Ayurvedic practice.

9.

Therapeutic Options: Panchakarma

According to Charka samhita, the body uses three routes to eliminate waste products and toxins: mouth, anus, and skin pores. The three doshas vehicle the ama either upwards to the Kapha dosha zone, downwards to the pitta or vata dosha zones, or to the periphery through blood vessels. The treatment of disease can broadly be classified as follows: ***Shamana chikitsa*** (palliative treatment) calms the vitiated doshas by appetizers, induced emesis, purgatives, digestives, exercise, exposure to sun, fresh air, palliatives and sedatives; this is a symptomatic treatment only. ***Shodhana chikitsa*** (purification treatment) involves internal and external purification to eliminate ama and mala in the body, followed by a cleansing process. ***Pathya Vyavastha*** regulates diet, activity, habits and emotional status to impede the pathological processes, to stimulate Agni, and to optimize digestion for assimilation of food for tissues strength. ***Nidan Parivarjan,*** or avoidance of disease causing and aggravating factors, is intended to proscribe precipitating or aggravating factors. ***Satvavajaya*** (psychotherapy) restrains the mind from desires for unwholesome objects, cultivates courage, memory and concentration. Although comparatively recent in the west, **psychology and psychiatry have been developed extensively in Ayurveda** and have wide range of approaches in the treatment of mental disorders.

Panchkarma (purification) proper is preceded by *Pre-purvakarma* regimen which requires sexual abstinence, letting go of natural urges, warm, comfortable and pleasant surroundings, meditation, and appropriate diet. The daily food intake should be light, nourishing and easily digestible, such as steamed vegetable and kichri which helps liquefy ama in the prapka digestion, calms the mind, is digested easily, and is highly nourishing. They are especially helpful in neurological disorders, musculo-skeletal disease conditions, certain vascular or neuro-vascular states, respiratory diseases, metabolic and degenerative disorders. Three pairs of approaches, six in total, are Reduction and Tonification, Drying and Oleation, and Sudation and Stambhana (Astringent methods). The first of each pair are meant to reduce excess factors in the body (obesity, hypertension) while the second of each pair are used for vata disorders as well as for low weight, low energy and improper growth of the body. Purification is attempted by **Vamana, Virechana, Basti** and **Nasya** and is the reverse of tonification for emaciated patients.

In **purvakarma** a patient is prepared to open channels, to liquefy the three humors by snehana (oleation) and swedana (fomentation), and to bring them into the digestive tract for elimination. **Snehana** saturates the body both internally and externally with herbal and medicated oils to stimulate the secretions in the dhatus, dissolves ama's sticky grip on dhatus, and reopens the shrota channels in each dhatu. Ghee is the best substance for internal oleation as it increases the digestive Agni without elevating cholesterol, reduces excess acidity, pacifies vata and lubricates tissues and joints, nourishes plasma and reproductive tissues, clears voice, and strengthens aura; sesame oil can also be used in place of ghee. Prescribed amounts of herbal ghee (generally 25-37.5 grams) are taken in the morning and the late afternoon on an empty stomach. The patient does not eat until the ghee is digested which is signaled by the return of appetite. However, heavy application of oils will depress Agni which can be rekindled by ginger and other spicy herbs. Animal fats (*vasa*) and bone marrow fat (*majja*) are also used sometimes in place of ghee for internal oleation. Both the internal and the external oleation are administered for seven days and success is signaled by a soft, shiny skin, yellow, shiny or oily fecal material, and ghee-like smell in both the urine and the feces.

Swedana or therapeutic heat is then applied to dilate the *shrotas* and for tissue expansion. Charaka mentions 13 different methods and implements to be used: saunas, steam, heated stone plates, herbal baths. **Nadi swedna** or penetrating heat from herbal water decoction is applied by a hose to the whole of body, and more particularly to the joints, for 5-7 minutes. *Bashpa swedana* or steam bath generally follows the **Nadi swedna**, with the aid of steam box that covers the entire body except the head which is kept cool by a compress; both procedures improve circulation. In other cases, poultice, dry heat, blankets, exercise, and herbal wines are used to apply heat. Swedana is not appropriate for people with heart disease and the patient should be kept hydrated by water intake. These two procedures are primordial for the success of Panchakarma as they move the toxins from dhatus and the doshas transport them back to the gastrointestinal tract.

Pradhan Karma or the main procedure consists of the five essential purification therapies: *Vamana* (emesis), *Virechana* (purgation), *Basti* (enema), *Nasaya Karma* (nasal cleansing) and *Raktamokshna* (bloodletting). Finally, *Paschat Karma* or follow-up therapies include diet, medication and lifestyle. *Panchakrma*-specific procedures may be directed towards kapha dosha (*vaman Karma, nasya Karma*), pitta dosha (*virechan karma, raktamokshana karma*) or vata dosha (*basti karma, anuwasan karma*), as the *doshas* perform their twice daily dosha gati.

Vamana. Emesis Therapy is really effective for nasal disorders, tuberculosis, bronchitis, asthma, diabetes, poor digestion, anorexia, dyspepsia, inflammation of lymph glands, epilepsy, insanity, edema, obesity, and heart diseases. Proper therapy brings about a feeling of cleanliness of the chest and stomach, lightness of the body and ensures timely passing of urine and stool. While over-administration could result in unconsciousness, blood vomiting, sudden drop of blood pressure and chest pain, under administration would not produce the desired effect. Therapeutic emesis uses herbs such as *yashti madhu* (licorice) and *madan phal* (*Randi dymotorum*) to dislodge ama out of the kapha zone, prevalent in all lung problems, bronchial asthma, allergies, chronic colds, rhinitis, diabetes mellitus, arteriosclerosis, arthritis, rheumatic diseases, and skin disorders like eczema, psoriasis and leukoderma. Contraindications are weak people, pregnant women, heart and blood pressure patients, patients with tuberculosis, pleurisy, hepatitis, and cirrhosis.

Vamana follows the seven day pretreatment with snehana and swedana, after the patient has shown signs of complete internal and external oleation. The night before vamana, the patient is given food which stimulates kapha: sweet, heavy, cool, sticky and oily foods such as milk, yoghurt, bananas and urad dal. Stomach secretions are stimulated by the herb called *vacha* (*Acoromus calamus*), generally in 1 gram amounts. Upon rising, the patient defecates and urinates, is given light snehana and swedana to increase body temperature for tissue expansion. The patient is now given about 300 ml of a thin, sweet-tasting porridge made from wheat and milk to promote watery secretions and increase the gastric volume. Some 355 emesis-stimulating herbs have been described but *madan phal* is most commonly used. The dried powder of the fruit is soaked in honey overnight and made into a paste of which one half tea spoonful is consumed by the patient along with a large quantity (1-3 liters) of warm licorice tea. Vomiting comes in bouts (generally 4-8) and is usually over in an hour; the expelled volume varies (325-1300 ml). The therapist should stand behind the patient to rub his back, sides, navel region and forehead. A sour, bitter, burning taste in the mouth indicates that the stomach is empty and the contents of the small intestine are now discharged. After 3-5 hours the patient receives thin rice water to rehydrate and rekindle Agni. Heart and blood pressure rates are monitored continuously as they normally rise during vamana.

Nasya. The nose is the gateway to the brain so it is important to keep the nasal passages and sinuses free of excess mucus and toxins. The administration of medicated oils through the nostrils is used to assist emesis therapy for dislodging toxins and excess kapha from the throat, nose, sinus and other organs. Nasya is indicated in diseases of the head and neck, for dry nasal passages, sinus congestion, common cold, chronic sinusitis, allergies and allergic rhinitis, headaches, migraine, epilepsy, eye and ear problems, and degenerative diseases. Dehydrated infants, pregnant women, and patients suffering from indigestion, thirst, hunger, grief or pregnancy, are not given nasaya. In excess it may lead to an excessive discharge from the nose and eyes, heaviness of the body, abnormal functioning of the sense organs.

In the first step, warm, herbalized oil is vigorously massaged on the face and the sinus area while the passageways are dilated using a hot, moist cloth or towel applied to the neck and face. Four drops of herbalized oil are then administered into each nostril. The herbs should have hot, pungent, dry and penetrating qualities to increase secretions that remove ama from the nose and head. The treatment is continued for seven days in a row and can be repeated for fourteen, and then twenty one days. Nasya for kapha, pitta and vata disorders are applied in the early morning, midday and late afternoon, respectively. **Shamana and bruhan** are palliative and nourishing types of nasyas that incorporate herbs (vacha and licorice) into ghee or sesame oil. *Pancheria vardhan* oil (Ashwagandha, pippali, naga bala and seven other herbs) is commonly employed and 8-15 drops are squeezed into each nostril. **Marsha nasya** and **prati marsha nasya** are milder procedures that use weaker herbs and 2-4 drops of oil every two hours. Nutritional nasya uses ghee, oil, salt in vata disorders, while sedative nasya uses aloe vera juice, warm milk, and gotu kala juice. Nasal massage consists of inserting the little finger dipped in oil or ghee into each nostril as deeply as possible and massaging gently to relax the deeper tissues. Calamus, bayberry, sage or ginger powder can be snuffed to clean the sinuses.

Virechana. Purgation therapy aims to eliminate the Pitta and Kapha which cannot be removed by emesis or through other channels such as the kidneys, lungs and sweat glands. It is highly effective in cases of fever, jaundice, skin diseases, bleeding from the mouth and nose, piles, worms, gout, vaginal diseases, anal problems, fistulas, anemia, glandular swellings and loss of appetite. It is not suitable for children, the old, the infirm and pregnant woman, and is to be strictly avoided under bleeding, weaknesses or diarrhea. It works downwards to eliminate pitta-related ama, such as hyperacidity, colitis, urticaria, acid peptic disease, hemorrhoids, chronic headaches, allergies and skin diseases such as acne, dermatitis, psoriasis, eczema, leprosy, leukoderma, and works on the digestive Agni in a dramatic manner. After snehana and swedana, the patient is given hot, sour and spicy foods that promote pitta secretions and virechana is administered 2.5 h later, performed either around noon or midnight. The medicine of choice is a decoction of Draksha, Aragwadha and Haritaki (12 g each) and Katuka 6 g, mixed with castor oil; some practioners use rhubarb, senna, aloe and Triphala in high doses. The patient has five to ten bowel movements within a few hours to expel 500 – 1600 ml fecal matter which is solid at first but progressively turns entirely liquid. Water with sugar cane juice and black salt is given to prevent dehydration and replenish electrolytes. The patient avoids, cold drinks, cool baths, and follows special diet for several days to rekindle Agni gradually.

Basti. The colon is the main organ of absorption of nutrients from prapka digestion, is the chief seat of vata, and constitutes the primary receptacle for waste elimination. Various segments of the colon are believed to be responsible for various diseases. Therapeutic rejuvenation of the colon is said to contribute 50% of the benefits of Panchakarma while all the other techniques combined together contribute the remainder 50%, as per Charaka, Sushruta and Vagabhata. Enema therapy is therefore effective for nearly all types of ailments in Ayurveda, as it helps to rejuvenate the body, purifies the colon, and permits control of the disease process before it goes into a migratory phase. Basti is most effective for vata related disorders, in the treatment of chronic constipation, low back pain, sciatica, rheumatism, gout, arthritis, neuromuscular disorders such hemiplegia, paraplegia, poliomyelitis, Alzheimer, Parkinson, multiple sclerosis, muscular dystrophy, epilepsy, mental retardation, and sensory dysfunction; contraindicated in colon disease, some forms of diabetes, diarrhea, and rectal bleeding.

Basti is administered only after oleation and sudation and consists of the introduction of medicated liquids into the colon through the rectum (***pakwashaya gata basti***); it can also be administered through the vagina (***uttara basti***), penis (***mutrashaya gata basti***) and wounds (***vranagata basti***) for specific dysfunctions related to those organs. External basti can be applied to the eyes (***netra basti***), lower back (***katti basti***), chest and heart area (***uro basti***), and head (***shiro basti***). Basti has also been classified according to its therapeutic function: ***shodhana basti*** (cleans and detoxifies); ***utkleshana basti*** (promotes secretion), ***shaman basti*** (palliative), ***lekhana basti*** (strong and penetrating), ***bruhan basti*** (nourishing), ***snehana basti*** (like anuwasan), ***rasayana basti*** (rejuvenation), ***vajikarana basti*** (for infertility), ***matra basti*** (for vata resulting from travel, exercise or stress). Charaka also describes three additional bastis depending upon frequency and duration: ***Karma basti*** is a month-long treatment for vata dominance; ***Kala basti*** is given for fifteen days to treat *pitta* dominance, and ***Yoga basti*** is given for eight days for kapha constitution.

Nirooha basti cleanses the entire body and uses a water based decoction of herbs given in 400-1200 ml amounts, 4-6 hours after the last meal in the morning or the evening. The concoction consists of ***dashmoola,*** made out of 10-15 herb roots, 30 ml sesame oil, a little honey, and a pinch of black salt; sometimes only one herb is boiled to ¼ original volume and 1 l is administered. This non-unctuous enema is followed several hours later or the next day, by 250 ml unctuous enema (milk+honey+oil+ghee), heated to 35 C. ***Anuwasan basti*** nourishes the body with the aid of herbalized oils and is given in 60 ml amounts in sesame oil. Nutritional bastis use meat broth, or bone marrow soup, while purgatory enema can be either oily or a decoction. All bastis are applied slowly but anuwasan is just a drop at a time, all prepared freshly. The patient is made to lie on the left side, extends his left leg, and bends his right knee towards the chest. This position makes the anal opening more accessible. Basti fluid is heated to near or at body temperature, drawn in a rectal syringe which is introduced 6 inches into the rectum using a rubber catheter, lubricated if needed, and the patient remains on his back for 10-20 min. In dehydrated patients, an oil basti precedes the cleansing basti. This procedure is repeated for eight to ten days and is always followed by anuwasan basti.

Raktamokshna. Toxins absorbed into the blood stream through the gastro-intestinal tract circulate throughout the body, so the purification of the blood becomes sometimes necessary. This therapy is very good in all imbalances of blood and pitta disorders and can provide dramatic relief in skin diseases, urticaria, rash, eczema, acne, scabies, itching and hives, tumors, gout, excessive drowsiness, alopecia, hallucinations, enlarged liver and spleen, hypertension, and some headaches. It is most often prescribed towards the end of the summer and during autumn when pitta is aggravated due to the dominance of Agni bhuta. It is contraindicated for infants, aged, those with anemia, edema, leukemia, internal bleeding, liver cirrhosis and pregnant women. Snehana and Swedana do not have to precede raktamokshna. A sharp scalpel is usually used to make superficial, parallel, or vertical incisions with extreme care after a soothing and antiseptic paste has been applied to the location; a needle can also be used instead. The amount of blood let out should not be more than 350 ml and leeches were used when smaller quantities had to be let out.

Paschat Karma (post-treatment rehabilitation) requires a graded administration of diet after panchakarma, starting with rice water ***(Manda)*** which is the first meal after vamana or virechana. Manda is just the plain water in which basmati rice was cooked, supplemented with ghee and a pinch of black salt. Thin rice soup (***Peya)*** is made from eight parts of water to one part rice and is followed by thick rice soup (**Vilepi**) four parts of water to one of rice. A little sugar cane juice and black salt can be added for taste. The fifth meal is ***odana*** or cooked rice while the sixth meal is *yusha* (lentil soup). The patient now gets *kichri* for a number of days but a normal meal may be possible after 6-7 intakes of the restricted diet.

Charaka proposes a number of panchkarma regimens or cycles.

1. Seven days of snehana, swedana and nasya followed by vamana on the eighth day and three days of samarajana karma after vamana.

2. Seven days of snehana, swedana and nasya followed by virechana on the eighth day and three days of samarajana karma after virechana.

3. Eight, fifteen or thirty days of snehana, swedana, nasya and basti.

One or two week programs are highly recommended once or twice a year for disease prevention, to be combined with *ritucharya* and *dinacharya* (chapter 13).

Massage and Acupressure

The literal meaning of 'massage' is **manipulation of the soft tissues** of the body using the hands. As a result of strong regulations in Europe and America, the most commonly practiced Ayurvedic treatments in the west are massage, diet and herbs. Safe and effective, it involves no pin-pricks, no heat fomentations, nor any chemical or electric stimulation. Massage is not recommended during fevers and pregnancy; abdominal massage should be avoided during diarrhea, ulcers, appendicitis, and abdominal tumors. It is customary for a **mother and baby to be massaged** every day **for forty days** after birth but the **child** continues to be massaged **until the age of three**. It makes the skin supple, controls vata by reducing its cold, dry, light, rough and erratic qualities, enhances blood circulation, encourages quick removal of metabolic waste and deep-seated toxins, improves flexibility as well as athletic performance and relaxes the body, alleviates pain, stress, sleeplessness and arthritic swellings. For general massage, the normal **direction of hair growth** is to be followed, a little extra oil is used over the body's vital parts; the scalp, head and the soles of feet are massaged once or twice a week. Sesame oil massage of soles and head at bedtime calms the mind and promotes sleep.

Oils are selected keeping in mind the therapeutic aim. Only bitter herbs are used and some 53 or more are decocted into a *tikta ghrta* (bitter ghee), according to the dosha constitution and digestive strength. General recommendations are: for pain, Narayan taila or Mahanarayan taila;

for weakness Narayan taila, Chandan Bala, or Lakshdi taila; for rheumatism Saindhavadi taila; for burning sensation and sleeplessness Bhringraj taila and Brahmi taila; for skin diseases, Kushthararakshas taila, Nimba taila and Bakuchi taila. Sesame oil is best for external oleation as it penetrates the skin, soothes vata without aggravating kapha and pitta, and promotes stability and strength but almond oil can also be used. The vegetable oils are sometimes supplemented with essential oils which are not retained by the body. The oil temperature should always be above the room temperature and the oil should stay on the skin for at least 15-35 minutes but can go up to 1 hour. Once the ghee and oil are absorbed, the excess is removed with gram flour (not soap). Peeli mitti (Indian yellow clay) is also excellent for washing the body as it cools the skin and nerves.

Vata massage is done with an excess of warm oils using smooth, firm strokes. The excess oil should be allowed to stand and soak into the tissue over the entire abdomen while the body is kept warm with sheets, pads and even blankets. Pitta massage is deep and varied but fast movement should be avoided for a calm and relaxing massage. Kapha massage requires vigorous strokes, with as little oil as possible, to stimulate their sluggish metabolism and fluid movement. Even fast, harsh movements are appropriate while the Kapha patient is drawn into a conversation. Oil to be used are sesame, coconut, mustard/sesame, respectively, for Vata, Pitta and Kapha constitutions. The oil bath is followed by a warm bath or shower but excess of soap and artificial scent are to be avoided.

Abhyanga massage is based on the principle of manipulation of crucial pressure points in the body. Numbering some 1000, these foci are actually small nerves about a centimeter in diameter and varying in depth between a quarter of an inch to several inches, often embedded in or near a muscle or a tendon. Massage begins with the upper limbs (arms), followed by the lower limbs (legs), chest, abdomen, back and hips, and ends with the face and the head; the massage **strokes are directed towards the heart**. However, it is a very exact art and should be carried out by a trained practitioner who knows the pressure points and applies correct pressure. Generally performed by two technicians, one each on either side of the body, massage can also be administered by one technician as the patient takes 30 different positions. Massage done by feet, used primarily in Kerala, is particularly good for athletes and its efficacy increases if the patient assumes yogic positions such as the *bhujangasasna*. **Filling the ears with oil** is a matter of course during every massage while the **eyes are soaked with ghee** which is permitted to remain for 333, 200 or 166 seconds, *for* vata, pitta, and kapha disturbances, respectively. Sometimes a patient is made to sit in a bath tub full of warm oil. Massage should always be followed by swedana (fomentation) to eliminate sweat and other waste products such as urine and stool. *Udvartana* massage is done with ointments and powders to remove oils applied during the Abhyanga massage. *Udgharshana* massage is done with dry herb powders to provoke heat and to open up pores and sweat glands.

Shirodhara is best performed after a general massage or *tarpana* as warm oil is dropped from a container 6-8 inches above the head, three inches above and between the eyebrows, for 20-30 min, followed by 30 min rest. The wick should extend 6 inches (15 cm) beyond the hole of the large pot and the stream should be as thick as the little finger. Warm oils are used for vata but cool oil is good for pitta and the prana vayu. The treatment is best done 7-10 AM on an empty stomach to calm the central nervous and care is taken to cover the eyes. *Shirobasti* is done by placing a leather cap on shaved head; the cap is filled with warm medicated oil for 53, 42 and 32 min, for vata, pitta, and kapha treatments, respectively; when the patient's nose starts to run, the treatment is successful.

Pischinchhali, from south India, uses vigorous massage with a bolus of rice wrapped in a cloth while large quantities of oil are poured over the body. It pacifies vata, stimulates the marma points, helps eliminate toxins, calms muscle spasms, and heals degenerative muscle disease. It must be administered many times in succession for about 30 minutes and is followed by *pinda swedana.* Here, rice cooked with special vata-pacifying herbs is wrapped into a pinda or bolus which is soaked in an herbal milk decoction of nutritive herbs. This hot bolus is rubbed over the entire body, focusing on muscle tissues and joints. It is usually performed after snehana for about 10-20 minutes. *Pinda swedana,* improves muscle tone and nourishes mamsa dhatu and vata. It is also highly beneficial for facial paralysis, hemiplegia, multiple sclerosis, and other degenerative diseases. *Tapa swedana or ruksha swedana* involves the application of sauna or hot sand to reduce inflammation and congestion in the joints. *Upanaha swedana* uses herbal poultice prepared with water and oil; the poultice is usually made up of *urad dal* cooked with herbs; it is particularly effective for gout, arthritis and inflamed joints. *Drava swedana* uses herbal decoctions in hot water as a hot shower or bath to enhance the effectiveness of the treatment. *Ushma swedana* uses steam applied either generally to the whole body or locally to the joints and marma points.

Kayakalpa is described in Siddha and Ayurveda medical literature as the ultimate fountain of youth, vitality, longevity, higher consciousness and *Jivan Mukti.* It goes back to thousands of years but was suppressed so severely by the British that few can perform it today. There were two types of Kayakalpa: The first method, **Kutipraveshika** (from "Kuti" or cottage and "Praveshika" or dwelling within), was a profound experience reserved for advanced Yogic practitioners who had the immense discipline needed to undergo the treatment. During 90 days, in a process of therapeutic austerity sustained by small amounts of a carefully selected nourishment, secluded in a three layered womb-like cottage protected from air and sunlight, the aspirant received special herbal-mineral elixirs and entered subtle states of consciousness that allowed them to rejuvenate completely. After determining the Ayurvedic type, a paste made out of 108 herbs was applied to the entire body while the patient maintained a tantric, connective breath. The skin was then brushed off and a shirodhara performed to create ecstatic sensations and expanded awareness. A hot bath using herbal extracts and aroma therapy was combined with **kundalini** stimulation to release unexpressed emotions and fears. Forgiveness released the patient from past projections and opened a new way to perceive relationships. The patient was then placed in a cocoon of sheets and blankets, the chakras were anointed with the most powerful essential oils while a deep meditative breath was maintained. The process continued over the next several weeks and even months.

The second method of rejuvenation, **Vatatapika** (from the Sanskrit Vata or air and **Tapika** or sunlight), was gentler and allowed the person to engage in the normal activities of everyday life. It was historically given to royalty who could not abandon their duties of state. Kayakalpa preparations are made from a wide variety of botanicals and minerals, ranging in composition from a single to 96 ingredients that had to undergo intensive purifications to break them up into very tiny molecules for quick assimilation. However, the body too had to be prepared to fully receive their remarkable benefits.

Surgical Procedures

Sushruta describes surgery (**shastrakarma**) as follows:

> *"Surgery is first and highest in the healing art, it is pure in itself, its use can never die, it is a product of the heavens and a sure source of renown on earth (to those who practice it)"*.

Sushruta details human anatomy along with more than 100 kinds of surgical instruments such as scalpels, scissors, lancets, needles, hooks, probes, detectors, forceps, syringes, specula, twenty types of steel knives depending upon their length and their qualities. He describes over 300 types of surgical interventions according to their use: **cheda** (incision), **bhedna** (excision), **lekhana** (scarification), **vedhana** (puncturing), *esana* (exploration), **aharna** (extraction), **visravna** (evacuation) and *sivana* (suturing). Experience was to be gained by different types of strokes using gourd, watermelon, cucumber, bamboo, quartz, glass, ruby, fire, caustic soda, and various leaves, cloth, stuffed dolls, scarification of plants, veins of leaves or dead animals, soft fruits, leather bags filled with water etc. Careful attention was paid to diet, climate, hydropathy, oral hygiene, and anointing the body before bath. Sterilization was practiced by fumigation, alkali and cautery. Anesthesia was administered using hemp, liqueurs, belladona and other products.

Surgery excelled that of **all other peoples and places** in the world and surgeons accompanied the army in Mahabharata. Bharata surgeons were reputed for **caesarian**, plastic surgery, skin transplants, cataract removal, hernia, dentistry, amputation etc., thousands of years before they became known in Europe. **Rhinoplasty** of the ancient Vedic-Buddhist tradition, lifting a flap of skin from the forehead to fashion a new nose, has **remained unchanged until today**. Sushruta mentions the **resection of the infra-orbital** plexus in case of neuralgia, laparotony and intestinal ligation in case of occlusion. Urine retention is described in specific hymns of Atharvaveda and Rigveda, to be relieved by breaching of the urethra and probing of the bladder orifice with an arrow like reed. This primitive catheter was described as *vasti-yantra* in later medical texts. Specific procedures were described to cater to such diverse disciplines as anatomy, embryology, toxicology and therapeutics. Fractures were consolidated with bamboo splints, a technique **subsequently adopted by the British** army as the "patent rattan cane split". Splinters (*salya*) were made out of wood, bone or metal but no mention is made of anesthetics though a little wine was recommended. Splinters were divided into fixed and loose, and fifteen methods are detailed for removing loose splinters. Blocked windpipe was cleared by the insertion of a tube in the throat which had been heated on a fire. Vedic surgeons even discovered sutures by ant bites whose mandibles formed clamps while the ant body was cut off.

It was recognized that the blood was pumped by the heart in all four directions, a **full 2500 years before William Harvey** was to establish it in Europe in 1628 CE. Bloodletting was used for prophylaxis against a range of skin disorders, alleviation of pain, clarity of mind, and reduction in the intensity of disease. Twelve kinds of leeches were described and Dhanwantari holds a leech in one of his hands in a tradition that goes back 5000 years, as leeches automatically separate from the body after sucking 10-30 ml blood. **Leech therapy later disseminated around the ancient world**, along with the rest of Ayurveda, and is making a comeback in modern medicine. In contrast, phlebotomy was used by Galen to treat plethora or an excess of blood in the body. Four ways were described to stop blood flow: closure, clotting, sepsis and cautery. Fifteen ways were described to mend split ears and ear piercing was also detailed.

Although Dr. Sir William Hunter had observed: *"The Surgery of the ancient Indian physicians was bold and skillful"*, to **justify colonialism** by a 'superior' race, European visitors to India from 17th century on spread the rumor that surgery was virtually unknown in India. In reality, all local medical knowledge was spread by the Buddhists from Central Asia to Philippines and transcribed in their respective languages so they now speak of a common heritage and westerners credit everything to the Chinese. **Vedic and Buddhist medical knowledge was to reach Europe** through the texts translated by Iberian Arab scholar Albucasis all of which influenced the Greeks and the Arabs. A policy was put in place where wrong translations deliberately ridiculed and belittled the original texts (chapter 1). Furthermore, **most Western scientists dismissed Ayurveda but also copied freely from it** (chapter 16).

10.

Yoga and Ayurveda

Yoga and Ayurveda are sister sciences; while Yoga connects the microcosm with the macrocosm, Ayurveda is the science of the body. Yoga aims to lift the individual, successively, from the physical sheath (***Annamaya kosha***) to the *pranic* sheath (***Pranamaya kosha),*** on to the mental sheath (***Manomaya kosha***), followed by the wisdom sheath (***Vijnanyamaya kosha),*** leading finally to the bliss (***Anandamata kosha),*** just as Ayurveda reverses the Samkhya creation leading to union with the macrocosm. Both share the same fundamental principles and look at human anatomy and physiology in the same manner. ***Hatha Yoga Pradipika*** includes oleation, sudation, enema and basti as part of the Yoga discipline while Ayurveda includes ***Yama*** and ***Niyama*** for rejuvenation. Specific Yogic asanas permit energy exchange between the panchamahabhutas, open and move prana stagnating in power centers as well as in ***nadis, dhamanis*** and ***srotas,*** clean the mind, body, and consciousness, and alleviate stress related diseases such hypertension, diabetes, asthma and obesity. Thus, the headstand grounds the intellectual activity and receives divine inspiration from feet pointing towards heaven. Lifting the legs brings earth to the head while touching feet with hands brings ether energy to the earth. In moving from one posture to another, one is moving through time and space until the Shakti and Shiva unite in the 7th chakra. Relaxation techniques like yoga, meditation, and prayer, work by changing gene activity responsible for response to stress. The very genes that are up and/or down regulated by stress, are switched the other way around during relaxation. Herbert Benson, at Harvard Medical School reported that over **2,200 genes** were activated differently in the long-time yoga practitioners, compared to the controls, and 1,561 genes were altered in the short-timers compared to the long-time practitioners (Times of India, 4 July 2008).

Patanjali was surely a great scholar of human mind as his 195 ***sutras*** are laconic aphorisms of the greatest scientific and philosophical ponderings. Part I on Meditation contains 51 sutras, followed by Part II on Practice and Part III on Accomplishments, of 55 sutras each; Part IV deals with Absolute Isolation and has 34 sutras. Part I is succinctly summarized by the first sutra where the essence of yoga is to oppose the tendency of the mind (*citta*) to run around. The practice of

Yoga (Part II) involves austerity, silent repetition of a mantra, and silent devotion to Ishvara, to control senses and attain a steady state in the mind. This is accomplished by the eighfold path of **yama, niyama, asana, pranayama, pratyahara, dharana, dhyana and Samadhi.** These have been further expanded as: Yama is ahimsa (non-violence), satya (truthfulnes), brahmacharya (sexual abstinence), atreya (non-stealing), and aparigraha (non-coveting, not desiring enjoyment). Niyama is tapa (austerity), japa (silent repetition of a mantra), santosha (contentment), sauca (physical and mental purification), Ishvarapranidhana (devotion to Ishvara or Purusha), svadhyaya (self study). Yoga postures (asanas) are meant to discipline of the body until they become as comfortable as the normal sitting position. Pranayama is breath control until restrain is spontaneous. Pratyahara is withdrawal of all senses. Dharana is concentration on internal space like the navel, plexus, third eye, tip of the tongue etc; Dhyana is a continuous state of dharana while Samadhi is meditation for oneness with the Universal. Part III describes siddhis obtained through yoga which endow unusual power over thought, speech, time, and space, and which are to be mastered to attain Part IV or fusion of the microcosm with the macrocosm. As all individuals have a part of divinity in themselves, by invoking the strength of that divinity through the control over ones thoughts, one can shape life. The way to control life is to control the choice of words and thoughts via relaxation, concentration, meditation, music and mantras.

Chakras, Kundalini, Marmas, Nadis, Dhamanis, Srotas

The main *nadis*, *Ida* and *Pingala*, run along the spinal column in a curved path and cross one another several times. At the points of intersections they form strong energy centers known as *chakras*. The Sanskrit word *"chakra"* means a "wheel or circle", or even a wheel of life. **The earliest mention of *chakras* is to be found in the *Upanishads*,** specifically the *Brahma Upanishad* and the *Yogatattva Upanishad*. The texts of *Agamas or Tantras* list 5, 6, 7, or 8 chakras but over time, the system of 6 or 7 chakras was adopted by most schools of yoga, largely through the translation of two Sanskrit texts, the **Sat-Cakra-Nirupana, and the Padaka-Pancaka.** Sir John Woodroffe, alias Arthur Avalon, in the book titled *The Serpent Power* and Zachary Selig in his book titled *Kundalini Awakening, a Gentle Guide to Chakra Activation and Spiritual Awakening,* have discussed these aspects in much detail. Some models describe one or more transpersonal *chakras* above the crown chakra, an Earth star *chakra* below the feet, and many minor *chakras* between the major chakras.

The notion of chakras was quickly amalgamated into many traditions such as *qi* (Chinese), *ki* (Japanese), *koach-ha-guf* (Hebrew), *bios* and *aether* (Greek, English), the *kabbalah* and *lataif-e-sitta* (Sufism and neo-platonism). Chinese practices like the acupuncture, itself 'borrowed' from Bharata, center around the energy *qi* which flows along the front torso channel, and enters the *dan tian* for union with Dao. According to the Himalayan Bonpo tradition, Chakras, as pranic centers of the body, influence the quality of experience, particularly if related to the heart and the throat chakras. In the Western hemisphere, a concept similar to that of prana can be traced back to Franz Anton Mesmer that used 'animal magnetism' to cure disease in the 18th century. Anodea Judith believes that chakra is a center of activity that receives, assimilates, and expresses life force energy. Susan Shumsky states that each chakra in the spinal column influences or even governs bodily functions near its region of the spine; the function of the chakras is to spin and draw in this energy to keep the spiritual, mental, emotional and physical health of the body in balance.

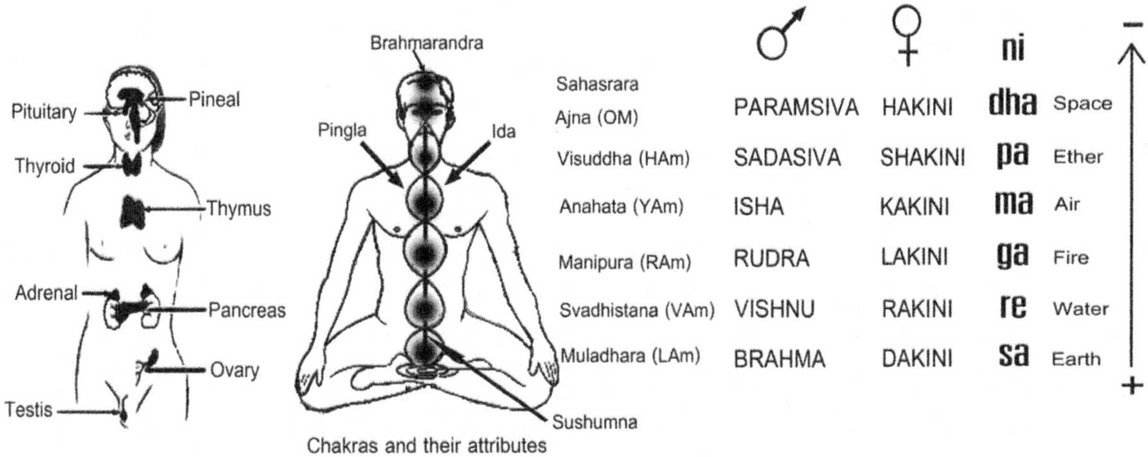

Figure 6. Chakras are related to the endocrine glands, the sound (shabda brahma), the male and female presiding deities of Tantra, the musical octave, the panchamahabhutas, and the electromagnetic spectrum.

In the original Eastern tradition, the chakras are thought to be psychic levels of consciousness and energy centers for the flow of prana; thus, 'proving' the existence of chakras is akin to 'proving' the existence of a soul. Paramhans Swami Maheshwarananda describes chakra as a powerhouse in the way it generates and stores energy. In Tantric texts the Sat-Cakra-Nirupana, and the Padaka-Pancaka, the chakras are described as emanations of a spiritual conscious energy from Brahman which gradually turns concrete, creating distinct levels of chakras, and eventually reposing in the Muladhara chakra. The energy that was unleashed during the creation, called the Kundalini, lies coiled and dormant in Muladhara. It is the purpose of the Tantric and Hatha yoga to arouse the latent Kundalini and make it ascend through the increasingly subtle chakras, until union with the universal is achieved in the Sahasrara chakra at the crown of the head (Figure 6).

Each chakra is visualized as a lotus with a certain number of petals related to the number of *nadis* that emanate from that chakra. The increasing number of lotus petals, in ascending order (though *Ajna* has only two), may be taken to indicate the rising energy or vibration-frequencies of the respective chakras, each functioning as a transformer of energies from one potency to another. Each chakra has its own geometric form, specific powers, control over senses (touch, taste, smell, hearing), elements (earth, air, fire, water, ether and space, i.e. progressively increasing volatility), sound vibrations, deities and *bija* mantra. There is a definite relationship between the musical octave **sa, re, ga, ma, pa, dha, ni,** and the chakras (Figure 6). Quantum physics says that the body is made up of energy and sustained by energy so the tendency since the 1940s has been to associate each one of the seven chakras with a given color and a corresponding crystal as per the spectrum **vibgyor**, from the most electronegative to the most electropositive; Mercier introduces the relation of color energy to the science of the light spectrum:

> *"As humans, we exist within the 49th Octave of Vibration of the electromagnetic light spectrum. Below this range are barely visible radiant heat, then invisible infrared, television and radio waves, sound and brain waves; above it is barely visible ultraviolet, then the invisible frequencies of chemicals and perfumes, followed by x-rays, gamma rays, radium rays and unknown cosmic rays".*

Associated with each petal is one of the fifty letters of the Sanskrit alphabet representing the vibrations produced on it by the Kundalini.Theosophical authors like C. W. Leadbeater and Johann Georg Gichtel, a disciple of Jakob Bohme, believe that chakras have a physical manifestation as well, related to the glands in the endocrine system, and nerve ganglia (plexuses) along the spinal column. The magnetic energy surrounding the body is called the aura and is created by the energy of the chakras. In **Surat Shabda Yoga**, initiation by an Outer Living Satguru (Sat = true, Guru = teacher) is required to reconnect the soul to the Inner Shabda Master (the Spoken Word) at the third chakra.

Muladhara or root chakra: color **red,** element **earth,** is located at the base of the spine, between the genitals and the anus. Although no endocrine organ is placed here, it is said to relate to the gonads and the adrenal medulla, responsible for the fight-or-flight response when survival is under threat. A muscle in this region controls ejaculation in the human male. Within this chakra resides the kundalini, waiting to be aroused and brought back to the source from which it originated. Muladhara is the base from which the 3 main psychic channels (nadis) *ida, pingala and sushumna,* emerge. It controls sexuality, lust, obsession, instinct, security, earth, survival, grounding, stillness and human potentiality, stability, sensuality; above all it directs smell, reproduction and excretion, and also the fear and the guilt complexes associated with them.

Muladhara is represented as a square *mandala* with **four petals** around a circle (the four corners of the world), that carry the sound vibrations letters VAm, SAm, SHAm, and SAm. The Bija mantra LA-m, silent LA, vibrating M, affects the upper legs and the anus. The innermost triangle is the *yoni* (vulva) containing the *Swayambu lingum* along with 3.5 coils of energy (sattava, rajas and tamas) which touch the back of a white elephant (Airavat of Indra) with seven trunks. The presiding God is the child **Brahma** with five faces or the five dimensions. He is granting boons, holding a *Danda* (staff) for body support, a *Kamandalu* (gourd) to maintain liquid balance, a *Rudrakshmala* of 108 beads and gestures *Abhayamudra* with the lower right hand to dispel all fear. The presiding goddess is **Dakini** (Kali) with four red hands dipped in blood, holding a *Sula* (spear) to symbolize the life target, a *Khatvanga* (staff with skull on top) to permit the rise of energy into the empty skull, a *Khadga* or sword for discrimination, a *Casaka* or drinking cup to fill the life with meaning. In Tantra, this chakra is equated with fuming of boiling sulphur, greenish-yellow, combining every repugnant smell, tasting rotten eggs, to be activated by rituals (see Frost).

Svadhistana or Adhishthana: color **orange**, element **water** is located in the sacrum (hence the name), just beneath the navel. It is related to sexuality, testes and the ovaries that produce sex hormones, the genitourinary system, and the adrenals. The Sacral Chakra is symbolized by a lotus with **six petals** that carry the letters BAm, BHAm, MAm, YAm, RAm and LAm. The Bija mantra VA-m (hard VA and relaxed M) is like the beating sea on a beach. Svadisthana governs action, reproduction, creativity, joy, enthusiasm, violence, pleasure, taste. Blockage of this chakra gives rise to emotional problems or sexual guilt. The lotus within the lotus is called the *Kunda* flower, while the *Ambhoja mandala* (crescent moon) represents water. The *makara* inside the circle is like a combination of an alligator and a fish.

It is presided over by the God **Vishnu** wearing a *Vanamala* or celestial garland, made out of forest flowers from all seasons and extending down to the knee. Vishnu carries a Chakra which symbolizes the mind, a *Gada* (mace or war club) to subdue the ego, and a *Padma* (lotus) to symbolize the spiritual goal. The four armed **Rakini** of blue color presides over the Svadhistana. She has three red eyes and protruding teeth to symbolize uncontrolled and uncultivated imagi-nation. She is holding a *Sula* (trident) to indicate the oneness of the mind, body and speech, a *Padma* (lotus) to point to the last chakra, **a *Damaru*** (drum) that represents mental talk and eter-nal time, and *Tarika* (axe) that symbolizes the battle of life. In Tantra, she is a woman in her reproductive mode in lustful rampage who wants more children, while a female spider is waiting for a male to impregnate her. Water roars here like the sound of an angry sea, smells bad fish, and tastes salty mucus, imbued with a pitiless emotion, while its vermillion-brilliant orange red is the virgin blood dripping from the yoni.

Manipura or Manipuraka: color **yellow**, element **fire**, is located in the solar plexus: linked to the Islets of Langerhans in the pancreas, and the adrenal cortex, that regulate metabolism, assimilation and digestion. This chakra is the seat of personal power, fear, anxiety, opinion-formation, introversion, and transition from simple or base emotions to complex. The **ten petals** of the lotus carry the letters DAm, DHAm, NAm, TAm, THAm, DAm, DHAm, NAm, PAm, and PHAm. The Bija mantra RAm (RA is deep in chest while M vibrates) corresponds with the animal ram representing strong emotions. The downward pointing triangle in the center circle is the Agni mandala with *swastika* marks on three sides. The presiding god is **Rudra**, or the male aspect of the unmanifest energy; he is holding a *rudrakshmala* to worship **Ishtadevata,** along with **Shakti** or fire weapon, while his gestures are granting boons and dispelling fears. Beautiful **Lakini** (Lakshmi) presides over the Manipura chakra, with three heads each having three eyes; she is holding **Vajra** (thunderbolts) as well as *Shakti* while granting boons and dispelling fears. In Tantra, she is full of possessiveness, jealousy and aversion, smells acrid sweat on a clean body, tastes cold like greasy mutton fat and rosemary.

Anahata or Padma-sundara: color **green**, element **air**, is related to the thymus in the chest which is linked to both the immune and the endocrine systems. It controls complex emotions, feel, touch, compassion, tenderness, unconditional love, equilibrium, rejection, well being, circulation, love for the self and others, passion, and devotion. The **twelve petals** carry the letters KAm, KHAm, GAm, GHAm, NAm, CAm, CHAm, JAm, JHAm, NAm, TAm, and THAm. The bija mantra Yam is extremely difficult to pronunce as there is some mathematical order behind it. The two triangles inside the circle point one each upwards and downwards. The animal antelope represents fleeting emotions. The *Kalpataru* (celestial wing tree) in the center of *Anandakanda* grants all boons, leading to *moksha* (salvation). The presiding god is **Ishah** (the male aspect of the unmanifest energy), the Lord of Speech. The attractive **Kakini** with three eyes and four arms presides over the Anahata chakra; she wears a necklace of bones, grants a boon and expresses fearlessness. She holds a *pasa* (noose) to remind you of your goal and a cup made out of skull containing the wine of life.

Vishuddha or Vishuddhi: color **blue**, element **ether**, is linked to the thyroid which produces thyroxin, responsible for growth and maturation, The **sixteen petals** of the lotus carry the letters Am, Am, Im, Im, Um, Um, Rm, Rm, Lm, Lm, Em, AAm, Om, AUm, AUm, AHm. The Bija mantra HA-m is sounded in the reverse manner from normal mantras, starts very low and gains power so that A overpowers H while the M vibration is louder than in most mantras. Vishuddha governs communication, growth, independence, fluent thought, security, creativity, communication, audition and speech. It is represented as a circle inside which is a downward pointing triangle containing the white elephant Airavata with six trunks (subdued will). It is presided over by **Sadashiva**, the male aspect of the manifest energy with five faces (omniscience, omnipresence, omnipotence, and sublimation of five senses), each face has a third eye of wisdom, 10 arms for efficiency and power, clad in a tiger skin, and a garland of snakes (wisdom). He carries *Pasa* (noose), *Arikusa* (goad), *Abhyamudra* (gesture), *Nagendra* (snake king), *Sula* (trident), *Dahana* (fire), *Ghanta* (bell), *Vajra* (diamond sceptre), *Krppana* (sword) and *Tanka* (battle axe). The friendly goddess **Shakini** (Gauri), mercy personified, presides over Vishuddha chakra, to drive you on with a whip, a bow and arrow, and even a noose; she is colored glistening light yellow, but is imbued with understanding to let you spiral higher. It symbolizes creation as an alert white elephant that can be molded as one will, smelling an open pine forest, tasting honey-sweet lemon.

Ajna: color **indigo**, element **mind**, is linked to the pineal gland which produces the hormone melatonin that regulates sleep and attention, as well as the psychedelic chemical dimethyltryptamine. The Bija mantra OM is the 13th vowel of Sanskrit which represents the life force, where the silent M persists eternally. The **two petals** carry the letters KSAm and HAm. Ajna balances the higher and lower selves and is related to the inner guidance, intuition, clairvoyance, psychic abilities, imagination, and dreaming. It is represented as a perfect circle containing a triangle which encloses the image of Yoni and a linga called *Itara*. A quarter moons and a bindu sign symbolize the essence of energy. The presiding God is **Paramashiva** and it is here that the yogis consciously place their prana at the time of death. The presiding goddess **Hakini** is both a creator and a destroyer. She has six heads, and her six arms are holding *Vidya* (book), **Damaru** (drum), **Khatvanga** (staff with skull on top), and **Mala** (rosary); while one hand is granting a boon the other is dispelling fear. There is no joy nor sorrow now as there is no need to be born again. In Tantra, this chakra is symbolized with the life force and represented by a ying-yang couple where a drop of crystal pure water is like the new seminal fluid.

Sahasrara: is the chakra of pure consciousness, perhaps related to the pituitary gland which secretes several hormones to integrate not only the entire endocrine system but also the central nervous system via the hypothalamus. Symbolized as a lotus with one thousand petals, it is located at the crown of the head and represented by the color **violet**. The **1000 petals** are arranged in 20 layers of 50 petals each. It has no element or bija mantra as such but AUM is sometimes used. It is related to the inner wisdom, death of the body, release of karma, universal consciousness, and "beingness". It has no presiding deities because all have fused into the macrocosm as prana escapes through **Brahmarandhra** at the very center of the skull.

Balancing the Chakras

Chakra work is neither easy nor painless but balancing is central to many different therapies and disciplines: hatha yoga, aromatherapy, mantras, meditation, reiki, laughter therapy, musicotherapy, hands-on healing, radionics, sound therapy, color/light therapy, crystal/gem therapy, to name a few. Furthermore, *marma acupressure, acupuncture, shiatsu, tai chi and chi Kung* all focus on balancing the energetic meridians that are an integral part of the chakra system, according to *Vajrayana* and *Tantric Shakta* theories. Some authors feel that it is best to open the chakras from the lower up. Sit in a comfortable position on a chair or on ground facing east and imagine a circle around the body inside of which you are protected, or simply request protection from higher powers while meditating. Now visualize a bright golden sun above the head whose cosmic energy is entering through the 7th chakra, down the spine through various chakras, the shoulders and arms, the hips and legs, energizing the whole being with light until it meets the earth energy rising up from the ground to the first chakra. Let the excess energy go back to the earth from where it came as the feeling of wellbeing permeates the body. Take a deep breath and imagine the golden energy surrounding and protecting the body.

1st Muladhara chakra: Sit in *padmasana* which brings the 1st chakra into direct contact with the earth and provides a good grounding effect. Wear red clothes and/or imagine a red glow around the 1st chakra permeating the whole body, awakening the senses, the fire and the passion in life. This chakra can be stimulated by aromatic oils from rose, jasmine, patchouli and sandalwood, massaged around the appropriate location. Gemstones recommended for this chakra are agate, garnet, bloodstone, black tourmaline, ruby, smoky quartz and hematite. Music with a steady, driving and forceful rhythm awakens the primal energy of this chakra while burning cedar incense calms the nerves. Yoga postures for Muladhara include: cobra, back stretch, spinal twist, cow face, and the corpse. The Divine Light Invocation will activate this chakra "*I am created, sustained, protected, surrounded, and ever growing into the divine light*". Imagine yourself and your bed surrounded by a divine light when retiring.

2nd **Svadhisthana chakra**: Imagine that the moon's nurturing beams are balancing the feminine energy of the second chakra. Wear orange clothes or imagine an orange glow around the 2nd chakra. Aromatic oils from bergamot, vanilla, bitter almond and sandalwood can be used to massage the appropriate area. Gemstones for this chakra include amber, carnelian, citrine, moonstone, gold topaz or calcite, and peach aventurine. Listen to the soothing type of music like the running water along with calming incense. Yoga postures for Svadhistana include the back stretch, cobra, plough, butterfly, abdominal curl, camel, and corpse. Practice the divine light meditation and fill the balloon-like, empty body with white energy till various limbs etc. fuse into one mass of white light, as described by Sivananda Radha.

3rd **Manipura**: Golden sunlight warms this chakra by contemplation on wheat fields bathing in the sun light and your favorite sunny meadows. Orchestral music with gong and brass sounds will relax the 3rd chakra. Wear yellow or imagine yellow light in the area of this chakra as this color lifts mood. Aromatic essential oils from lemon, acacia, lavender, rosemary and bergamot can be used to stimulate and balance the Manipura. Gemstones for this chakra include amber, aquamarine, carnelian, citrine, emerald, gold, malachite, perridot, pyrite, smoky quartz, topaz. Yoga postures for the Manipura chakra are the spiral twist, abdominal curl, mountain, tree, back stretch, and corpse.

4th **Anahata**: Imagine a stroll in the countryside with beautiful wild flowers, green and lush fields. Listen to classical and sacred music, wear green clothes or imagine green light near the heart for inner peace, new growth, and serenity. Massage with aromatic oils from mint, sage, musk, tuberose, ginger and rose will activate this chakra. Gemstones for Anahata include carnelian, jade, ruby, malachite, emerald, rhodochrosite. Yoga associated with Anahata is bhakti or devotion to dissolve the ego into the ultimate reality; postures to activate the 4th *chakra* include: mountain, lotus, bow, cobra, fish, shoulder stand, and corpse.

*5th **Vishuddha***: Imagine a blue sky and its reflection in a body of water; sense the peace, calm and the magnificence of the bubbling ocean. Music and songs rich in high tones and choral music will stimulate and cleanse the 5th chakra. Wear blue and imagine blue light activating this chakra in the throat area. Aromatic oils used to calm, cool and cleanse the 5th chakra include eucalyptus, myrrh, lilac, sage, and oregano flowers. Gemstones recommended for Vishuddha are aquamarine, azurite, blue lace, agate, topaz, sapphire, lapis lazuli, and turquoise. Chanting of mantras like AUM will activate Vishuddha. Recommended yoga postures include: spinal twist, sun salutation, lion, cobra, head and neck rolls, and corpse. Meditate on light; imagine a lotus bud at the base of the spine and a spark of light emerging from it, going up the spine all the way up to the pituitary and the pineal, and down back to the very first vertebrae.

*6th **Ajna***: Contemplate on the starry, deep blue night sky as you listen to the classical and sacred music. Wear indigo blue and imagine a beam of indigo in the forehead on or near the area between the eyebrows. Massage the chakra area with aromatic oils from lavender, gardenia, mint, rosemary and jasmine, all of which activate the senses and increase awareness of surroundings. Gemstones for Ajna include amethyst, sapphire, topaz, lapis lazuli, tourmaline, and quartz. Jnana yoga and Tantra yoga are associated with the 6th chakra while beneficial hatha yoga postures are: back stretch, mountain, shoulder stand, lion, sun salutation, palming the eyes, and corpse. The Divine Light meditation and a hollow spine filled with White light are combined with correct breathing where white light is drawn in during inhalation and with every exhalation the light is focused at the desired level of the spine. *Mahamudra* is practiced regularly as well.

*7th **Sahasrara***: Imagine being alone on a mountain top and feel the presence of an omnipresent spirit around you. Any music that enhances the inner silence will be good, as will the mantra AUM. Wear violet or white clothes which contain all of the colors of the spectrum and imagine a violet light shining on the top of the head. Massage the scalp with aromatic oils from lotus, clove, peppermint, and cinnamon. Gemstones for the 7th chakra include amethyst, diamond, rock crystal, serenity, and emetine. Recommended yoga postures are spinal twist, sun salutation, the tree, rubbing the tip of the head, head stand, and corpse.

Nadis and Kundalini

The word *nadi* comes from the Sanskrit root *nad* meaning "channel", "stream", or "flow" from Chandogya Upanishad. Nadis are sometimes viewed as extending only to the skin of the body, but are often thought to extend to the boundary of the aura as well. Nadis are not nerves or arteries but rather channels for the flow of consciousness. Just as the negative and positive forces of electricity flow through complex circuits, in the same way, ***param shako*** (vital force) and ***manas shako*** (mental force) flow through every part of our body via these nadis. Nadis are thought to carry a life force energy known as ***prana*** in Sanskrit, or ***qi*** in Chinese-based systems. In the Western traditions and Interpretations, the three main nadis (***Ida, Pingala and Sushumna***) are sometimes related to the Caduceus of Hermes:

> *"the two snakes which symbolize the kundalini or serpent-fire which is presently to be set in motion along those channels, while the wings typify the power of conscious flight through higher planes which the development of that fire confers".*

In this framework of mystic western esotericism welded with yoga concepts, sometimes the three nadis are related and named as alchemical sulphur and alchemical mercury:

> *"In the East, the symbol of the two serpents twisting on the rod corresponds to the two currents Pingala and Ida which coil around the Merudanda: the first is red, hot and dry, likened to the Sun and the Alchemic Sulphur; the second, Ida, is cold and wet, like the Alchemic Mercury and is correlated with the Moon for its silver pallor"*

The ***Sat-Cakra-Narupana*** explicitly refers to three main nadis, named ***Sasi, Mihira,*** and ***Sushumna*** but in some tantric texts more than 72,000 nadis are cited. Ancient manuals describe upto 350,000 nadis through which the prana flows. The six most important are: ***ida*** (surya), ***pingala*** (chandra), ***sushumna, brahmani, chitrani*** and ***vijnana.*** Ida, pingala and sushumna originate at the base of the spine and travel upwards. While ida and pingala criss cross each other as they travel up via the spinal column, sushumna divides into anterior and posterior portions at the level of larynx both of which terminate into the ***brahmarandra.*** The junctions of ida, pingala and sushumna form the chakras from where nadis radiate outward to other parts of the body. In the average individual, prana flows through ida and pingala but sushumna stays blocked at the first chakra where the latent prana lies dormant as kundalini.

The Ida and Pingala nadis are often referred to the two hemispheres of the brain. The word pingala means "tawny" in Sanskrit, equated with solar and male energy. Pingala courses from the left testicle to the right nostril and represents the river Yamuna. It is seen as red, of positive polarity, and corresponds to the left side of the brain. Pingala is the extroverted (active), solar nadi, and corresponds to the right hand side of the body and the left hand side of the brain. The word ida means "comfort" in Sanskrit, Ida is the introverted, lunar nadi, and corresponds to the left hand side of the body and the right hand side of the brain (crossing occurs at the optical chiasma). Ida has a moon-like, female energy with a cooling effect, is of a pale color, negative polarity, and refers to the right hand side of the brain. It courses from the right testicle to the left nostril and corresponds to the river Ganges. Ida nadi controls all the mental processes while pingala nadi controls all the vital processes. The Nadi Sushumna, whose substance is the threefold gunas, is in the middle. She is like the Moon, Sun, and Fire; her body, a string of blooming *dhatura* flowers, while the Vajra inside her extends from the Medhra to the Head.

The nadis are approached through the corresponding nostrils, stimulated through different types of Pranayama, e.g. the alternate breathing from left and right nostrils which would alternately stimulate the brain. Although asanas were not elaborated upon by Patanjali, they were performed to train the body to remain still without effort. The rhythmical breathing and special breathing techniques are supposed to influence the flow of energy in these nadis. The breathing techniques will purify and develop the energetic currents and will lead to special breathing exercises to awaken kundalini. In *Raja Yoga* of Patanjali, when the mind has been calmed through Yama, Niyama, Asana and Pranayama, the important state of Pratyahara begins where dispersion of mind ceases. This is characterized by observing the movements/jerks in Sushumna which connects the base chakra to the crown chakra, from the perineum to the juncture of the lamboid and sagittal sutures of the cranium.

Kundalini is sometimes compared to a coiled serpent whose activation can release energy for spiritual transformation. When kundalini is awakened, she uncoils and begins to rise upwards like a fiery serpent, breaking upon each chakra as she ascends, until Shakti merges with Shiva in *sahasrara chakra*. Typically, the energy release begins in the lower part of the body and moves upwards. Kundalini travels through the Brahma nadi at the centre of sushumna which is enveloped by the chitra nadi. As kundalini pierces each chakra, that lotus opens, and as soon as she leaves for a higher chakra, the lotus closes its petals and hangs down, symbolizing the activation of the energies of the chakra and their assimilation into kundalini. This ascent through the chakras can be viewed as an upward journey through the self which refines and subtilizes the energy of the kundalini. Although spontaneous arousal can occur at any age, **Hatha yoga awakens *kundalini* by purifying the *nadis*,** disciplining the body, tonifying the nervous system, and regulating the flow of prana by kriyas, mudras and bandhas. Awakening of the Kundalini leads to the attainment of psychic powers or eight *siddhis*: ***Anima*** (power to assume a minute form), ***Mahiman*** (power to assume an extensive form), ***Gariman*** (power to become weighty), ***Laghiman*** (power to become light), ***Prapti*** (power to reach the most distant objects), ***Prakamya*** (power to obtain what is desired), *Isita* (power to shape anything) and *Vastiva* (power to control anything). All of these must be mastered to attain Nirvana, the final union with the ultimate reality where Being finally fuses with the Non-Being.

Marmas

Marma means secret, hidden and vital, and represents the connection between the physical body and the subtle energetic centers. Marmas or lethal points in the body are junctions where the **flesh, bones, sinews, pipes, ducts and junctions converge**, and where the life prana is most concentrated. As sensitive zones, marmas can hold various emotions like fear (vata), anger (pitta) or attachment (kapha), the three gunas sattva (calm), rajas (aggression) and tamas (inertia), as well as prana, tejas and ojas. In fact, the concept of marmas goes beyond modern medicine and its purely mind-body relationships. They serve as 'pranic control points' on the body, where the energy of prana can be treated, controlled, directed or manipulated in various ways. They form the **very basis of Acupuncture.**

The 107 marma points are grouped according to the region of the body: 22 each on the upper extremities and the lower extremities, 12 in the abdominal and chest regions, 14 in the back and 37 in the neck and head. They have also been classified based on the structure: muscles 11, blood vessels 41, ligaments 27, joints 20, and bone 8. If injured, 9 cause instant death, 33 cause death in time, 3 cause death if hit by a foreign body like a bullet, 8 cause pain, and 44 cause disability. Certain marmas, touched in a specific manner, can confuse, incapacitate, paralyze, and inflict pain or disability. Traditionally, marma points are grouped into 3 categories: on the legs and feet, (*Sankha marma*); on the trunk (*Madhayamanga marma*); on the neck, and on the head (*Jatrurdhara marma*); *Kshirpa* marmas at the extremities of hands and feet can be stimulated to alleviate the diseases of the corresponding internal organs. While many marmas are at the surface of the body, like points on the hands or feet, others are internal like the heart and the bladder. The head has the greatest concentration with special marmas governing the eyes, ears, nostrils, mouth and brain. Yet marmas can also be found along the front and back of the trunk as well. The pulse itself is one of the prime 'vessel' (*shira*) marmas in the body, where the patient's energy can be read and understood. Besides these primary marmas some authorities mention up to 360 non-physical marmas, located in the sphere of prana around a person, in the aura, certain points above or behind the head, and sensitive points on the body. The skin itself can be regarded as a greater marma zone in which all the other marmas are contained. The chakra points at the top of the head (*adhipati marma*) or the third eye (*sthapani marma*) are important marma points as well. Similarly, the end points of various nadis on the palms, the soles, the corners of the eyes, ears or nostrils are important marmas. Marmas vary in size from one finger length or digit (the most common) to four finger lengths or about the width of the hand. Marmas in turn are related to the chakras, nadis and srotas.

The main aspect of Yoga that actively considers the use of marmas is Pratyahara, which mediates between the outer factors (Asanas and Pranayama) and the inner factors (Meditation) of Yoga. In ancient Vedic times, marma points were called ***bindu*** – a dot, secret dot or mystic point. Like a door or pathway, activating a marma point **opens into the inner pharmacy of the body**. The body is a silent, universal, biochemical laboratory, operating every moment to interpret and transform arising events. Touching a marma point changes the body's biochemistry and can **unfold radical, alchemical change** in one's makeup. Stimulation of these inner pharmaceutical pathways signals the body to produce exactly what it needs, including hormones and neurochemicals that heal the body, mind and consciousness.

Marma Therapy

Marmas are important diagnostic as well as therapeutic points, used to balance the doshas, to increase Agni, to reduce ama, to promote energy (***vajikarana***), and aid in rejuvenation (***rasayana***). **Marma-point massage dates back to southern India circa 1500 BC** both as part of Pancha Karma and daily self-care. For example, massaging marma points on the head, like those around the eyes, ears, nostrils and mouth, is an important way to stimulate one's mind and senses in the morning. Marma therapy is particularly good for arthritis and other structural problems, as well as for treating any type of nerve pain or paralysis. Therapeutic pressure points or Marmas are of five types: ***Mans marm, Sira marm, Snayu marm, Asthi marm, and Sandhi marm***, where vital energy or prana is locked up.

Ayurveda treats marmas more so with massage, acupressure, oils and aromas, than with acupuncture. Medicated oils or tailas, herb exracts in a sesame oil base, are used for specific forms of massage where two technicians, one on each side of the patient, apply a series of perfectly synchronized, directional strokes on the back and the front of the body that match the vata's five different directions that control all physiological functions (chapter 7). They are massaged with the thumb over an area as large as six inches across in small, gentle, clockwise circles moving outwards and then back inwards, slowly increasing pressure and area of the massage circle.

Acupressure consists of about five circles going out and five coming back, three times each. Aroma therapy is another important tool for treating marmas, either with massage oil or inhalation, because aromatic oils have a strong ability to influence prana and alter energy. Stimulating oils like camphor, eucalyptus or cinnamon are used for opening up energy at marma points, while cooling and sedating oils like sandalwood or khus serve to calm or consolidate the energy. Applying camphor, menthol or eucalyptus to the marmas on the nostrils to remove congestion is one such a stimulating marma therapy, while applying cooling and calming sandalwood oil to the third eye to treat headaches is a sedating approach.

While much of marma therapy consists of massage and direct touch, another significant procedure involves energy treatment or pranic healing, in which touch may be light or even indirect. Here, the prana of the healer is as important as the physical manipulation of the marmas. This can be compared to the martial arts in which a master with a strong qi or prana can stop or knock down an opponent with his own energy, using only a light touch or no touch at all. **Dhanur Veda** trains a warrior how to recognize marma points as well as the different blows that can be used to affect marmas in various ways to harm the enemy. Chinese and Japanese martial arts, wrestling, gymnastics and *t'ai-ki k'iuan* improvise marma manipulation, first **developed in ancient Bharata**. An Ayurvedic healer with a good prana can have a strong healing effect by his prana alone, even without using any significant touch or physical manipulation. This more subtle or sattvic form of touch is often best for treating the mind, emotions and deeper consciousness of the person.

Dhamanis and siras. Sushruta mentions 24 Dhamanis and 700 Siras, responsible for respiration, defecation, menstruation etc, but their precise locations have stirred controversy. It is now clear however, that the 24 Dhamanis correspond to the 24 meridians of acupuncture consisting of 10 ascending (**Dhatu Dhamani**), 10 descending (**Ashaya Dhamani**) and 4 transverse (**Tiryag Dhamani**). Embedded into these channels are the external marmas and 700 siras. There are four types of siras, of which the 40 original provide points to eradicate disease by puncture, pressure etc. These 40 original siras are called **Vatvaha, Pittavaha, Kaphvaha, Rakyavaha**; each is subdivided into 175 as they reach **vat-sthan, pitta-sthan, kaph-sthan and rakta-sthan**, respectively. Sushruta says that it is the **rasa** (Chinese Qi) that **flows into dhamanis and not blood**. This rasa is responsible for life support 24/24 hours. Rakta mokshan does not mean blood letting but the revival of the speed of circulation of blood. The meaning of one **Prastha Shonit Mokshan** does not mean removal of 13.5 pals of blood but the time required to stimulate the **Sirabindu** = 13.5 minutes. Certain Siras should not be needled but acupuncture or **Agnikarm** at the right point permits smooth circulation of rasa (Prana) and blood. Specific details are provided as to the weather, timing, site selection, instruments, depth of insertion (2.5 mm above the bones and 5 mm in the muscular areas), duration and frequency of acupuncture.

Srotas. Ayurveda sees the body composed of innumerable channels that supply the various tissue. Srotas are a network of 22 channel systems which permit undisturbed flow of life force. They are not situated in the regular channels like the Dhamani and Siras but are more directly related to the main organs. **Pranavaha srota** carries prana and is situated in the cardiac and pulmonary regions but its action also extends to the brain. Vata, Kapha or Pitta imbalance can dysregulate this srota to be treated by warm oil massage of **Sthapani marma** at the level of the third eye, and the **Talahridya marma** at the center of plasma and soles, combined with alternate nostril breathing and meditation. **Annavaha srota** carries food and is situated in the esophagus and stomach; the related disorders can be treated by correcting jatharagni using Trikatu, chitrak and cayenne, along with massage of Indra Basti marmas on mid lower arm and the mid-calf regions. **Ambhuvaha srota** carries water and is situated in the palate and the pancreas; its dysfunction gives rise to diabetes. **Udakavasha srota** is situated in the hard and soft palates and regulates the corresponding water metabolism; its dysfunction can be treated by massage of **Basti marma** between umbilicus and the pubic region, as well as of **Urvi marma** in the mid upper arm and mid thigh regions. Herbs like punarnava, gokshura and lemon grass give excellent results. **Rasavaha srota** carries blood and is situated in the heart and blood vessels, as well as the lymphatic system, and controls blood and food circulation whose disorders are to be treated with massage from clavicule down to the sternum on the front, and circular massage on the abdomen. **Raktavaha srota** carries blood and is situated in the liver and spleen, vitiated by an excess of Pitta, and treated by blood purifying herbs like manjishta, turmeric, burdock, prawal bhasma (coral oxide) and Moti bhasma (pearl oxide). Masage of **Hridya marma** and of the twelve marma points in the throat region (eight **Sira Matruka marmas** and two **Manya marmas**) should also be considered. **Mamsava srota** supplies mamsa or muscle; it is situated in the muscle and skin and its dysfunction can be treated with vata pacifying drugs along with blood purification. **Astivaha srota** supplies asthi and is situated in the adipose tissue around bones and buttocks whose dysfunction can be treated by Vata pacification through massage of **Sthapani** and **Adhipati** marmas. Colon disturbances can be controlled by massage of **Shankha marma** in the temples and **Utkshepa marrma** just below it. Diet should contain natural calcium like the oyster shells and sesame seeds along with enemas of sesame oil or milk containing ghee, shatavari and ashwagandha. **Medovaha**

srota supplies medas and is situated in fat tissue around the kidneys and abdomen whose dysfunction can be treated with herbs like guggul, myrrh, cyperus, chitrak, and black pepper; *Guda marma* should be massaged in obese patients. *Majjavaha srota* supplies majja; it is situated in the long bones and joints and transports cerebrospinal fluid whose vitiation is to be treated with nervine stimulants (gotu kala, jatmanasi, shankhapushpi) along with massage of the five *Simanta marmas* in the cranial sutures and the four *Sringataka marmas*; *Sthapati and Adhipati marmas* are to be treated by shirodhara. *Shukravaha srota* supplies shukra and is situated in the testes and penis for the transport of semen, to be treated with kayakalpa rasayans, vata pacification, and massage of *Guda* and *Kukundara marmas*. *Svedavaha srota* carries sweat and is situated in the adipose tissue and skin for the transport of sweat whose dysfunction is to be treated with oleation, sudation, diaphoretics (cinnamon). *Purishavaha srota* carries feces and is situated in the anal canal and the rectum for the transport of stool whose dysfunction (diarrhea or constipation) should follow the corresponding therapies. *Mutravaha* srota caries urine and is situated in the large intestine and the urinary bladder for the transport of urine; dysfunction is to be treated with diuretics (purnava and gokshura) along with the massage of *Katika, Taruna* and *Kukundar marmas* as well as with *Basti marma*. *Artvavaha srota* carries menstruation fluid and is situated in the uterus and the fallopian tubes that can be dysregulated by Pitta and Vata vitiation and Apana vayu; to be treated with herbs like saffron, turmeric, motherwort, valerian and jatamanasi and the same marma points as for the urinary system. *Stanyavaha srota* carries breast milk and is situated in the breast and the nipples for the control of lactation that can be disturbed by an increase in vata and kapha; to be treated with shatavari, licorice, sesame seads, cyperus, fennel, dill, and dandelion. *Manovaha srota* carries thought in the mental system.

Some of these channels have been **visualized by electron microscopy** only in recent years. Their existence **in Ayurveda, thousands of years ago**, is a tribute to the great meditative powers of the rishis and **no comparable description** is available in any **other system of medicine**. Colonial powers did their best to ridicule these concepts, as they could not be visualized with the tools then available, and now some of this knowledge is being **patented as accomplishment of the European stock**. With this trend, the original discoverers could well remain buried in the anonymity of manuscripts gathering dust in the forgotten archives of libraries.

11.
Pranayama, Meditation and Mantras

Pranayama

Prana is the vital energy of the universe: *pra* = first unit, *na* = energy and *ayama* = expansion, extension or restraint. *Prana* is controlled by the voluntary regulation of inhalation, exhalation, and the pause between them; in Sutra 1:34 Patanjali uses different words for these processes. Three types of breathings are possible. In **diaphragmatic inhalation**, air is taken in by contracting muscle fibers to move the diaphragm downward which decreases the volume of the abdominal cavity but increases that of the chest. Physiologically, this is the most efficient type of breathing. In **chest breathing**, the diameter of the thorax is expanded via the intercostals to expand lungs and air is pulled in to fill in the newly created space. This chest breathing expands the middle and upper portions of the lung, but is not so efficient with the lower portion and is also less efficient than the diaphragmatic breathing. The chest breathing requires more work for gas exchange than does the diaphragmatic breathing and also needs more heart work for pulmonary circulation. Most people employ a variant of either chest or diaphragmatic breathing. The **clavicular breathing** expands the uppermost part of the thoracic cylinder to create more capacity at the very top of the lungs. The **Yogic complete breath** incorporates all three: it is initiated by the diaphragmatic contraction thus oxygenating the lower lung fields; the middle parts of the lungs are then expanded with outward chest movement in the thoracic phase; the clavicles are finally raised to expand the uppermost part of the lungs. Other types of breathing result from autonomic control during 'fight or flight' response and the ensuing hyperventilation can cause irritability or anxiety. **Paradoxical breathing** involves a combination of chest expansion simultaneously with the contraction of the abdominal muscles, and stems from shock or surprise. In sleep apnea, associated with depression, decreased sexual drive, and confusion, breathing can stop for periods up to one minute with definite detrimental effects on health.

A Yogi counts his **life span as the number of total breaths**. We breathe 18,000 to 20,000 times every day and the internal nose is closely connected to the brain, the pituitary, the limbic system, the olfactory nerve and other strategic structures. Freud was conscious of the interaction between the reproductive organs and the nose; menstrual cramps were often related to nasal inflammation. Diet determines the composition of the nasal mucus whose consistency is related to either resistance or susceptibility to infections, allergy, hay fever etc. The shape of the nose affects the manner in which prana is supplied to the body and the brain. Breathing predominates for 100-120 minutes each through either the left or the right nostril. Ancient yogis had realized that having the left or the right nostril open would gear us toward one type of activity or another. Right nostril breathing was associated with alertness in the external world while left nostril breathing produced a quieter psychological state. Food digestion was favored by keeping the right nostril open before eating while passive fluid intake was done with the left nostril open. Sinuses are cavities that are adjacent to, and open into, the nasal cavity, and also secrete mucus. Inflammation pulls in blood, mucus and fluids into the sinuses leading to sinusitis. Tears produced by the lachrymal glands also drain into the sinuses. *Jalaneti* with saline solutions at body temperature is very effective in clearing sinuses. Here, water through one nostril is permitted to come out of the other. In *sutra neti*, a rubber catheter is taken in through the nostril and taken out through the mouth.

Pranayama cleanses the lungs, heart and other organs and purifies the nadis but if done incorrectly it will produce disease. Therefore, it is important to get help from an experienced teacher. It is a process through which one can isolate the inner self from mechanical thought process, control emotions, induce calmness, alleviate nervous disorders, refine sense perceptions, awareness, concentration, extra sensory perception, etc. It permits control over the mind itself by the triple process: ***puraka*** (inhalation), ***kumbhaka*** (retention) and ***rechak*** (exhalation) and its practice increases alpha waves in the brain. Pittas should inhale left and exhale right for cooling effect; kaphas should inhale right and exhale left; vatas should do alternate nostril breathing. Yoga manuals recommend that one lie on the left side after meal, open the right nostril to stimulate digestion, and to increase body heat. The obese should perform the 'breath of fire' exercise where a deep breath is exhaled quickly. It should be done for one full minute followed by one minute of rest, another minute of exercise, for a total of 10 minutes. A 16 min program can include 3 minutes of alternate nostril breathing, 10 minutes of sun salutation and again 3 minutes of alternate nostril breathing.

To harmonize breath, lie down on the back and place a hand each on the chest and the edge of the rib cage where abdomen begins. The abdomen rises during inhalation and falls during exhalation with relatively little movement of the upper chest. Next, rhythmic diaphragmatic breathing is combined with slow inhalation to bring more air and nutrients into the air sacs and blood stream. This is done in shavasana (corpse posture) while exhaling completely through both nostrils, followed by inhalation, and minimizing the pause. A variant is to put a 5-10 pound sandbag between the chest and the abdomen in shavasana so diaphragmatic breathing can be experienced without any effort. In Makarasana or crocodile breathing, one lies flat on the stomach, hands on the biceps such that the chest does not touch the floor, to initiate the diaphragmatic breathing; during inhalation one feels the abdomen pressed against the floor and during exhalation one feels the abdominal muscles relaxing

Nadi Shodhanam (alternate nostril breathing) requires a prior mastery over complete yogic breath. The right nostril is closed with the right thumb followed by completely exhalation through the left; the left is then closed as one inhales through right; total of three equal exhalations and inhalations complete one cycle. In more advanced forms, the ratio 1:4:2 is used for inhalation, retention and exhalation, respectively. Retention of breath after exhalation is later on added to the retention after inhalation. Whereas shodhanam without retention can be practiced safely, retention requires the guidance of a teacher. At first, 12 inhalations and 12 exhalations, without retention, are done to complete one round. Advanced stages follow 4-16-8 sequence; close right nostril with the right thumb, exhale through the left nostril to the count of 4, close the left nostril with the ring and the little fingers, hold to 16, open right nostril and exhale to 8. Now inhale through the right nostril and repeat the process in reverse. In more advanced stages, meditate on the sound A during inhalation through the left nostril, on the sound U during retention to the count of 16, and on the sound M as during exhalation through the right to the count of 8. The inhalation is now done through the right and the process is reversed. Sometimes, one concentrates on a mantra: **ha** is the sun (right side) and **tha** is the moon (left side).

Kapalbhati (lustrous forehead and face) pranayama cleans sinuses and stimulates the abdominal muscles along with the digestive organs. This entails a vigorous and forceful expulsion of breath using the diaphragm and abdominal muscles, followed by relaxation of the abdominal muscles, resulting in a slow, passive inhalation; to start with eleven expulsions are performed in each round. ***Bhastrika*** is similar to Kapalbhati but both inhlation and exhalation are forceful, repeated in quick succession, starting with 7-21 cycles, 20 inhalations and exhalations are performed, to a total of 20 bhastrika rounds. *Ujjayi* (control or victory) breathing enhances lung ventilation, removes phlegm, and vitalizes the whole body. Here, both the inhalation and exhalation are slowed by partial closure of the glottis during inhalation; the ratio between inhalation and exhalation is 1:2. Retention is then performed with *Jalandhara bandha* (chin lock) while both nostrils are closed. During inhalation, the incoming air is felt on the roof of the palate accompanied by the sound *sa* which is felt as *ha* during exhalation. In *Bhramari* (buzzing of the bee) pranayama, air is inhaled through both nostrils; a humming sound is produced during exhalation as in *Ujjayi*; repeated for 2-3 minutes. Both *Sitali* and *Sitkari* cool and soothe the body. The tongue is curled and protruded outside the lips in the former and retracted back to the palate in the latter. Inhalation makes a hissing sound followed by complete inhalation through both nostrils; repeated three times each. In *Suryabhedana*, breath is inhaled through the right nostril, retained and exhaled through the left. In *Plavini* (float on water), the stomach is filled completely with air, the lungs are then filled to capacity, the breath is retained and then exhaled slowly. In *Kundalini pranayama,* attention is focused on the *Muladhara chakra* in the alternate nostril mode. Imagine drawing in prana with left inhalation to the count of 3 AUMs, send down the current through the spinal column to the count of 12 AUMs, and exhale right to the count of 3 AUMs. Prana healing is done by concentrating on the light flowing into the body, never out of the body, which is visualized as a channel for the healing light. Here, the Mantra *So ham Hamsa* can be used along with the Divine Light Invocation.

Breath retention should not be practiced without applying the bandhas that lock the prana in a certain area. In *Jalandhara bandha,* glottis is closed while gentle pressure is applied to the chin by pressing it against the chest to produce a trance like condition and blissful state of mind that slows down the heart. When the jalandhara bandha is not applied, the inhaled air wants to rush out through the auditory tubes and produces various disorders in the inner ear. In *Mulabandha,* the anus sphincter muscles are contracted and held during pranayama and meditation; various mudras are applied as well e.g. *jnana mudra, Vishnu mudra.* **Mudras permit the energy to flow in only one direction** instead of alternate paths. It is equally important to assume a comfortable posture e.g. Sukhasana, Swastikasana, Siddhasana, Padmasana, Maitriyasana, and Vajrasana. The idea is to **develop breath awareness**: flow, noise, pause between inhalation and exhalation, shallowness etc without which awakening of sushumna is impossible. Eventually, the **breath should start flowing** freely and smoothly in **equal measures through both nostrils.** Some yogis need less than one breath an hour.

Meditation

According to Swami Vishnu Devananda, meditation is *"….a continuous flow of perception or thought, just like the flow of water in a river"*; by constant observation of the mind it permits **control over the internal world** to discover the wisdom and tranquility that lie within. Meditation brings awareness, harmony and natural order into life; it is ideal for disciplining the mind and removing stress and strain after the bath in the morning to bring harmony and natural order. Critical in satisfying the mind's hunger, when done well it is so nourishing that the body can survive on less. **Control of desire**, or mental hunger, is the **key to longevity and immortality**. *Ahmakara* (ego) due to pride, anger, delusion, greed, jealousy, hatred and lust, is the root of all bondage and meditation creates positive channels by effacing *samaskaras* engraved on the mind. Diet and sexuality should be controlled and **silence** cultivated as it is the **language of God**. Whatever thought or deed comes from a person will return to him in some form or another. Every thought vibrates through the mind, provoking electrical and chemical changes. Brain waves in EEG consist of *beta, alpha, theta* and *delta* waves, corresponding to consciousnesses, normal waking, altered consciousness and deep sleep, respectively. Experience meditators can emit brain waves of 30-40 micro-volts, (normal man = 15) in the *beta* zone while advanced yogis have recorded outputs exceeding 100 microvolts. Meditation does not add any new powers but only awakens the dormant ones, reduces the need for sleep, improves anabolism, reduces catabolism, and rejuvenates all cells with positive vibrations. The merging of the individual into the cosmic consciousness brings Samadhi. Meditation proceeds in **five stages**: argumentative, requiring an object with shape, size etc; non-argumentative, the object loses its qualities leaving behind only the form; deliberative, or the subtle essence of the object; non-deliberative, beyond space, time, and free from memory, word or meaning; the fifth and the final stage is without seed and all impressions are destroyed.

Some recommendations for meditation are: 1) Have a special place and specific time for meditation, preferably dawn (**brahmamuhurta**) or dusk, facing north or east to align with the magnetic vibrations. Enter this area only while meditating; soon this area will acquire vibrations to calm you down. 2) Sit up straight with your back, neck and head in one line, in a relaxed posture, regulate breath e.g. three seconds each of inhalation and exhalation. 3) Regulate breathing; start with 5 minutes of deep breathing then gradually slow it down. Follow a rhythmic breathing pattern - inhale and exhale. 4) Concentrate on your thoughts, desires and emotions, let them wander, and then slowly bring them to rest on the object of your choice. To cleanse yourself of distractions and increase awareness, observe your breathing which is the movement of prana. 5)

Focus on an object of your choice e.g. sun and its golden color, a candle, an image, flowers, fruits, trees, the sign AUM, until the object persists at the ajna chakra or the anahata chakra even when you are not looking at it. 6) In candle gazing, look at the candle in a dark room and then close the eyes until an after-image of the bright flame persists. In frontal and nasal gazing, concentrate on the 'Third Eye' at the tip of the nose, start with one minute and increase it to ten minutes. In *Yoni mudra*, close the ears with thumbs, eyes with the index fingers, the nostrils with the middle fingers; the lips are pressed with the remaining fingers. Release the middle fingers gently to inhale and exhale as you meditate. 7) Hold your object of concentration at this focal point throughout the session. 8) Subsist only on fruits and milk.

Mantras

The Bible observed: *"In the beginning was the Word, the Word was with God, the Word was God"*. In *Brahmanagrantha* we are told nine times that: *"Word is God, the speech is God, whatever is speech is God, God is the supreme space of speech"*. According to **Shabda Brahma** (speech), attributed to Bhartrhari 450 CE, *"The Word-Principle is Brahman; God itself…The purification of the Word is the very siddhi, attainment of God, the Supreme Self"*. Speech (*vac*) is the feminine principle of the universe sent by Prajapati to be transformed into various objects. In the Vedic age and later, linguistics, grammar, etymology and related sciences were so integrated and perfected that they have not been excelled even now anywhere in the world. Patanjali says that Panini wrote his linguistics while in meditation in a super conscious state. Panini grammar is based on 14 **Shiva sutras** (aphorisms) such that the whole **Matrika** (alphabet) is abbreviated by **Pratyahara**. Sanskrit grammatical tradition **vakarana,** one of the six *Vedanga* disciplines, began in late Vedic Bharata and culminated in the **Astadhyayi** of Panini, which consists of 3990 *sutras* (ca. 5th century BC). A century after Panini, Katyayana composed **Vartikas** on Panini *sutras*. Patanjali, who lived three centuries after Panini, wrote the *Mahabhasya*, the "Great Commentary" on the Astadhyayi and Vartikas of Katayana.

Patanjali defines **sphota** (from **sphut** or to burst) as the invariant quality of speech. The noisy element (**dhvani**, audible part) can be long or short, but the *sphota* remains unaffected by differences in the individual speaker. Thus, a single letter or 'sound' (**varna**) such as k, p or a is an abstraction, distinct from variants produced in actual enunciation. This concept has been linked to the modern notion of phoneme, the minimum sound needed to define semantically distinct sounds. Patanjali's objectives were metaphysical, to permit correct recitations of the scriptures

(*Agama*), maintaining the purity of texts (*raksha*), clarifying ambiguity (*asamdeha*), and also for the pedagogic goal of providing an easier learning mechanism (*laghu*). This strong metaphysical bent has also been indicated by some as one of the unifying themes between the Yoga Sutras and the Mahabhasya. The first fourteen *sutras* of Patanjali simply enunciate the letters of the alphabet, considered mothers of the universe by Tantra because of their vibrations. The Sanskrit word *shikshah* simple means phonetics whereas there is no logic of sounds in the western languages; the **Europeans learnt their phoetics through Sanskrit**. As there are no alphabets in Chinese, mantras were written in the *siddham* script but later translations corrupted the mantras.

In the Tantric view, the causal vibration or the **Shabda Brahman is the soundless Sound** which is aroused by a primal shudder and splits the Shakti into the female Nada and the male Bindu forces. The alphabet is the differentiation of the very first sound at the time of creation but differentiation continued until fifty articulate sounds were formed which combined to give rise to the visible universe. The deepest aspect of this science deals with the **place of the letters in various chakras**. From different concentrations of energy in the chakras, various syllables burst forth into the mind. All **vowels are feminine** while all **consonants are masculine**. The vowels (feminine energy) need no support in order to be articulated but consonants need vowels to be articulated. The seeds of all sounds exist in AUM, and **all vowels are variations of the primary vowel *a*.** Thought, form and sound are all the same just as steam, water and ice are the same substance. This process occurs in four stages: *Para* (the transcendental sound) is God where the diversity is unmanifest, *Madhyama* (thought transcribed as words) is speech where manifestation is diversified, and *Pashyanti* is the fusion of divine knowledge into soul and individual spirit through kundalini; *Vaikhari* (dense spoken word) is speech as inspired mentation. In *Tantrashastra* by Abhinavgupta in 11th CE Kashmir, the **colors in meditation** arise as the letters of the mantras **touch their natural origins** in consciousness. Special Tantra dictionaries give meanings and synonyms of each letter of the alphabet.

Hymns and mantras were deified as Brihaspati whereas **speech** was similarly deified as *Vac*. Sanskrit (well formed) words were the sound forms of objects, actions, and attributes related to the corresponding reality, perceived by the ear in the same way as visual forms are perceived by the eye. Thought was considered internalized speech. The elitist tradition of the priesthood separated ritual texts from secret teachings passed on from one generation to the other as correct pronunciations and incantations. Only Brahmans knew this speech to perform sacrifices, much as gods had done to reach heaven and Creation in Vedic hymns is described as the work of a divine craftsman via a fire sacrifice. The **Purusha sukta** or the "Hymn to the Person" (Hymn to the Primeval Man) states a careful correlation between the sacrifice and the universe. The basic identity of the Purusha or the universe is defined first, followed by a systematic correlation of various features of the universe with the sacrifice. The conception is very similar to **Vac** or Speech:

> *"The three quarters that are set down in secret they do not bring into movement. The fourth quarter of Holy Utterance is what men speak".*

Speech is man's most constant expression, the foremost tool for self-expression, and a way to relate the self with others. In Rigveda vac or speech is compared to a cow with abundant milk and mantras are considered more purifying than the waters. So, words must be chosen carefully because the power of words is not different from the power of thoughts. Because a word communicates your thoughts, choose words for their content of *sattva, rajas* and *tamas*. Devi mother *Shakti* is the goddess of the spoken word and her four attributes are: **Mahesvari** (wisdom), **Mahakali** (strength), **Mahalakshmi** (harmony) and **Mahasarasvati** (perfection). The words man, mind, mental, are all derived from the root **man** in Sanskrit which means to think, to contemplate, to meditate. The ancient *muni hymn* in the Rigveda states:

> *Drunk by what proceeds by silence we flourish on the airs, pranas; You mortals merely see our physical bodies.*

Bhuta Vidya is based upon chanting or sound therapy, called mantra in Sanskrit, composed by using specific vowels and consonants. Hindu and Buddhist religious practitioners believe that the repetition of **mantras links them with deities**, and yields supernatural powers which can be used to cure many diseases. The priests of different eastern religious sects transmit the Mantras to their devoted disciples during special ceremonies. The practice of spiritual healing, related to the activities of priestly lineage, has never broken its ancient spiritual connections. The traditional priest families of Nepal, India etc still claim to have good reputations for their skills as spiritual healers. Mantras are phonetic vibrations of the underlying fifty eternal sound oscillations of the Sanskrit syllables whose tremendous energy can be released by chanting of mantras aloud or silent. The **pronunciation is all important** here as the correct vibration wavelength leads one back through time to the **original vibration**, or the Supreme Power. As sound energies that have always existed in the universe, they cannot be created or destroyed and command the power to heal one physically and spiritually. Mantras help one to concentrate in meditation and when the mental processes have been exhausted through the chanting of a mantra, the mind becomes open to very subtle, intuitive perceptions. An electric field is created by the chanting of mantras where voice and emotions must work together. Vibrations can be felt in the body of people who have chanted mantra for say three hours.

A mantra has many levels of meaning and is composed of *nada* before they become letters. In Level A, **so** equals the inhaled and **ham (hum)** the exhaled breath sound. In level B, the sound cycles are heard as *hamso* and the meanings become clear so = he or that, aham = I; I am he or I am that. In Level C, the question is followed by the answer in a cycle: *soham* becomes *hamso* which sounds continuously in every living being; the heart repeats it 21, 6000 times over 24 hours. Only the most adept understand the meaning of *hamsah* for it represents the Sun of life force with which the yogi identifies himself and becomes parama hamsa. In Level D, **hamsah** means **sah**: body or prakriti permeated by the indwelling spirit **ham**. In Level E, the kundalini rises from the **sa (sam)** in the lowest chakra to arrive at the **ham** in the sixth chakra, having moved through all of the 50 Sanskrit letters, and the yogi now fuses the garland of letters in the 7th center into a single, universal sound. Tantra states that there are sixteen progressively advanced stages in the refinement of mantra.

For over 5000 years, the secrets of mantras and sounds were passed on from the guru to the disciple through **bhuta lipi** which is a coded sign language such that the vibrations could be maintained and it could not be understood by laymen due to several layers of meanings. Guru is *gu* = darkness, *ru* = to remove, he who removes darkness. Initiation means rebirth from the womb of the guru. Mantra given by an unqualified teacher can lead to problems with prana and kundalini. Always authenticate the tradition of the initiator who is moved by compassion and indebtedness to his own guru, and who has no material expectation from his student. Manu gave 38 mantras to his youngest son to be found in Book X *suktas* 61 (27 mantras) and 62 (11 mantras) of Rigveda, though the authorship is attributed to Nabhanedishtha (son of Manu). Manu is the first human being and is equivalent to the Hebrew and Arabic Nuh as it is always a Manu who leads e.g. after primordial floods; Manu intervals have been mentioned in texts on astronomy. During the Vedic age, spiritualism so pervaded the daily life that the spiritual laws were applied at every step. **A person who had a mantra became a mantra.** Acceptance of mantras in the west will transform life just as the numerals had done 13th-15th century CE.

Every mantra must fulfill several conditions: 1) it was originally revealed to a sage, 2) it has a presiding deity, 3) it has a specific meter, 4) it possesses the bija or the seed, 5) a plug conceals the pure consciousness. Specific mantras have specific powers but the Gayatri mantra is the supreme mantra of the Vedas and its repetition 125,000 times secures the grace of the presiding deity. *Nirguna* or abstract mantras are without form that set up powerful vibrations in the body, while in *Deity* mantras a specific form is visualized along with the repetition of the sound. For example, when the name Shiva is repeated with concentration, the sound actually breaks down one's lower qualities, the energy dances like *tandava*, in keeping with the quantum theory, until the name, form, and self are indistinguishable. In *Saguna mantras*, the Deity is the Mantra itself as the visible portion of the sound; a **translated mantra is no longer the body of the deity**.

In *Bija mantras* the **name is merged with the sound** and the mantra itself is the subtle body of the deity that acts directly on nadis, vibrates the chakras, and activates the kundalini which pulsates with the vibrations of the fifty basic sounds that reach gross articulation through the vocal chords. Bija mantras belong to no language, have no gender, no delineation, and personify the relationship between the kundalini and the Supreme consciousness. The original mantra AUM is the root of all sounds, letters, language, and thought; it represents the universal soul where the lower part of the symbol (female energy) signifies the diversity of the universe, pronounced as the sound Au, while the upper crescent signifies the universal reality (male energy) with the sound of nasalized M. All mantras are hidden in AUM which is the universal symbol of shabda Brahman, or God. The universe comes from AUM, rests in AUM and dissolves in AUM. This all pervading sound can be heard by yogis as all letters of the alphabet emanate from AUM where A= physical plane, U = astral and M = deep sleep state. Proper chanting requires breath control through pranayama. The 'Au' is generated deep within the body, from inside the navel, and slowly brought upward joining with the 'M' which then resonates through the entire head. Correctly pronounced, the sound moves up from navel to the nostril; the larynx and palate are the sounding boards, no part of the tongue or palate is touched. The cosmic sound AUM has one male (**hum** during exhalation) and one female (**so** during inhalation) component. If **all of the sounds could be recorded simultaneously**, one will obtain the eternal sound **ooooooooom-mmm**. Chanting in a whisper correctly for twenty minutes relaxes every atom in of every cell of the body and invokes pure, supreme vibrations. To hear the sound of AUM is the crown of all spiritual experience which means the ability to surrender. The panchamahabhutas have their own bija mantras: HAM, YAM, RAM, VAM, LAM (ether, air, fire, water and earth, respectively); these are not given to the initiate and are used with intricate rituals. Other bija mantras are: HAUM (Sadashiva), DUM (Durga), KREEM (Kali), HREEM (Mahamaya), SHREEM (Maha Lakshmi), AIM (Saraswati), KLEEM (Kamabija or Kamadeva), HOOM (Shiva/Bhairava), GAM (Ganesha), GLAUM (Ganesha), and KSHRAUM (Narasimha).

Vibrations in the sounds of names are attuned to cosmic vibrations. The moon, the sun, the twenty parts of the horizon, and the twelve signs of zodiac are all states of breath associated with a given syllable. Swamis receive a new name, as do wives and sometimes men after marriage. A new child's name was decided according to the letter that falls within the movement of the moon and a new Yoga initiate could be given a new name according to the position of the moon at the time of initiation. After initiation, nuns and monks are given a sacred name. The music is a product of the inner consciousness of an accomplished person who then gives it *dhvani* (sound) so the world can hear it, just like the speech we make. **Tanapura produces the undifferentiated cosmic sound nada** which is divided into inner sonar vibrations called mantra before being expressed as dhvani. In fact all **Indian music was an attempt to reproduce the inner sounds heard by practioners of Nada Yoga**. The word namah occurs in many mantras derived from the word *nam* "to bend" or "to salute" but Yoga tradition says *na mama* means "not mine" used in **namas te**: *"I hereby give up all claims of my ego in your honor. I adore and worship the Deity who is within you"*. Mantras are chanted with correct pronunciation for prolonged periods of time until the cosmic energy overwhelms the practioner.

Japa, or repetition of mantra, bestows the virtues and powers of the Mantra's presiding deity and destroys mental impurities. It is done with the aid of a mala (garland of **Sandal or Rudraksha**) of 108 beads, plus the Meru bead, and is never allowed to hang below the navel. The **fifty letters of the alphabet were divided and subdivided to correspond with the 108 parts of the universe**. Holding it in the right hand, start at the **meru** and roll the beads along one by one between the thumb and third fingers while repeating the mantra. After reaching the meru, the mala is rolled in the opposite direction because the meru bead is never to be crossed over. The most authentic mala of 108 beads plus one was originally made by virgins in Brahmin families, a gayatri mantra was repeated for each knot; when they reached the top further mental observances were required. Upon completion, the mala was taken through special sacraments, dipped in holy water while incense was burned. Some rudraksha seeds have five faces that correspond to the five aspects of special **shivamantras**. The **number 108 may also correspond to the 36 x 3 cycles of nadi-shodhan** in the morning, noon and evening. Rudraksh mala is also called the Varna mala where syllables are joined by the thread of breath passing through them. The movement of the mala in hand is used to release tension and is sometimes placed in a sack called **gomukhi**. Japa can be **vaikhari** (audible), **upamsu** (whispering or humming), and **manasika** (mental) which is the most powerful. It is done generally 20-30 minutes every day while the beads are rolled and the image of the chosen deity is visualized around *ajna* or *anahata chakras*. A concluding prayer and reflection on the deity end the session but mental japa can be continued throughout the day. In audible repetition, correct pronunciation is of primeval importance. Some scholars suggest that, of the 50,000 or so Sanskrit speakers in Bharata, less than 1000 are able to pronounce mantras correctly. The humming of Brahmins, while conducting a *hawan* ritual, is totally ineffective and such ceremonies have no beneficial effect whatsoever. It is therefore better to proceed with mental repetititon, especially for people of foreign origin who can barely pronounce Sanskrit. **Likhita mantra,** or writing, is another form of japa, done for 30 min with complete silence and concentration. Over a long period of time, deity *mantras* are repeated 100,000 times for each syllable of the mantra to complete one *puraschara*.

12.

Complementary New Age Therapies

Over the past ten years, the attitude in western countries has undergone a remarkable change regarding alternative therapies of the east which were all but shunned during the race dominated colonial era. However, some Christian and Muslim groups are against Yoga and many therapies related to it. The rationale behind most, if not all, of the alternative medicines stems from the nature of chakras that can be awakened and balanced by a number of factors (chapter 10). **Pilates** was developed in the early 20th century by Joseph Pilates in Germany to tonify the entire body by proper alignment, concentration, control, precision, breath, and movement, based on aerobics and yoga postures of Suryanamaskar. As of 2005, 11 million people practiced Pilates in the United States regularly, with the aid of 14,000 instructors. **Stretching** is a form of physical exercise in which specific skeletal muscle(s) is deliberately elongated to its fullest length in order to improve elasticity and reaffirm muscle tone. All of these stretching positions, some with artificial aids, are **essentially basic hatha yoga** under a western label. Many sports clubs offer **'Modern dance'** where the subject moves gracefully from one yoga asana to another, without maintaining the posture for any length of time.

Aromatherapy

Smell is **ten thousand times more sensitive than taste** because the olfactory nerve directly connects the limbic system of the brain to the external environment. Animals use smell to select their fodder and people reject food that smells rancid or otherwise spoiled. Man has the capability to distinguish 10,000 different smells. When the receptor cells in the nasal cilia receive the aromatic molecules, a signal is sent to the olfactory bulb and then on to the limbic system and hypothalamus. While lavender aroma increases alpha waves in the back of the head, associated with relaxation, Jasmine increases beta waves in the front of the head, associated with an alert state. The aroma of calming oil would release serotonin, and elicit a sedative brain wave pattern while a stimulating aroma causes an alert response. The tender yellow flower of the Ylang Ylang tree is considered so worthy of love that it is placed on wedding beds in Indonesia.

The story of **perfumes in Bharata is as old as the ISC, going back to 5000 BC**. Integrated into daily life, scented plants were used to celebrate every aspect of culture, from the ritual to the culinary, from the celibate to the erotic. With the passage of time, scented oils were extracted by pressing, pulverizing or distilling aromatic vegetable and animal produce. Such processes led to the development of the art of alchemy, the earliest indications of which are available from the **perfume jars and terracotta containers** of the Indus Valley civilization. The word 'attar', 'ittar' or 'othr' is an Arabic word which means 'scent', derived from the Sanskrit word *Sugandha*, meaning 'aromatic'. The **earliest distillation of *ittar* was mentioned in Charaka Samhita** and archeological excavations have revealed round **copper stills for making ittars that are at least five-thousand years old**. These stills are called *degs* and traditional ittar-makers, with their degs, traveled all over India to make fresh ittars on-the-spot. Even now, a few traditional *ittar*-makers travel with their gear to be close to the harvest. In ancient Bharata, ittar was prepared by placing precious flowers and sacred plants in water or vegetable oil. The plant and flower material would release their aromatic essential oils which could then be concentrated as ittar. The first ittars to be made were Rose and Hina. Ittars may be broadly classified according to the flavor or the ingredients used.

Floral ittars are manufactured from single species of flowers: Gulab (*Rosa damascena*), Kewra (*Pandanus odoratissimus*), Motia (*Jasminum sambac*), Gulhina (*Lawsonia inermis*), Chameli (*Jasminum grandiflorum*), and Kadam (*Anthoephalus cadamba*). **Herbal Ittars** are manufactured from a combination of floral, herbal and various forms of Hina: Shamama, Amber, Musk, Amber and Musk Hina. Some ittars are neither floral nor herbal. While alcohol (common solvent for most perfumes) causes the perfume to evaporate very fast, the oil-based ittar is worn directly on the body as a small drop. A few drops can also be added to water and used with aromatic vapor lamps, or with cold drinks to give fragrance. Ittar has a permanent shelf life and some ittars become stronger and smell better with age.

Essential oils are made up of alcohols, aldehydes, ketones, phenols, terpenes, sesquiterpenes, ethers and esters, all of which protect the plant against bacterial, viral or fungal invasions. A single oil can contain hundreds of constituents which exert various effects on the body. These oils are present in all parts of the plant albeit in varying concentrations. They are extracted either by steam distillation, cold pressing, CO_2 hyperbaric production, or solvent extraction, but steam distillation is by far the most preferred method because such products grow richer with age and may even have unlimited life span. It can take up to 2000 pounds of rose petals to produce one pound of rose essential oil through distillation, while lavender flowers yield essential oils in the ratio of 50 to 1. Consequently, the prices vary by a factor of hundred to one, or more. Altogether, some 150 essential oils are known all of which are light sensitive and must be stored in dark, glass bottles. Essential oils are quickly absorbed by the skin and reach lymph and blood systems from where they can be taken up by different organs and tissues, but **leave the body within 48 hours**. Lad and Frawley have defined essential oils as: alterative (restore normal health), antipyretic, antispasmodic, aphrodisiac, astringent, tonic, carminative, diaphoretic, diuretic, emetic, emmenagogue (regulate menstruation), emollient, expectorant, haemostatic, laxative, nervine, rejuvenative, sedative, stimulant, vulnery (assists in wound healing). Ittar oils are free from alcohol and any preservatives or chemical additives. However, fresh herbs have the most complete healing properties, dried herbs and essential oils are a close second choice.

Ayurveda classifies the energetics of each herb and oil into drying or moisturizing, and warming or cooling. **Warm Ittars** like Musk, Amber, Kesar (Saffron), and Oud, are used in winters to increase body temperature. **Cool Ittars** like Rose, Jasmine, Khus, Kewda, Mogra, are used in summers and cool the body. This fits in very nicely with the notion of chakras with red, electro-positive, hot (*yang*) at the bottom and blue, electro-negative, cold (*yin*) at the top of a vertical line. The electro-negative at the top have extra electrons and take heat away from the body while the missing electrons in the electro-positive produce heat as they gain electrons. While wet oils have high polarity and mix well with water to produce a moisturizing effect, dry oils are lipophilic and produce a drying effect. An oil that is hot and wet would correspond to pitta energetics while an oil that is cold and wet would correspond to kapha energetics; an oil that is cold and dry will correspond with the vata energetics.

Ayurvedic **blending avoids using opposites** as one oil will negate the effects of the other. One of the most common ways of blending is based upon the evaporation rates. Top notes evaporate fast and constitute 10-15% of the total blend. Middle notes form the 40-80% of the body of the blend. Base notes, also known as fixatives, comprise no more than 5% of the blend, fix or hold the smell by slowing down the evaporation rates. Carrier oils can be as important as the essential oil; sesame and hazelnut oils are best for vata while olive or sunflower, and sweet almond oil or mustard, are best for pitta and kapha, respectively. Aloe Vera oil is good for all types of doshas. Blending is done after detailed consultation to **balance the doshas**. Oils are used sparingly as large doses reduce effectiveness and can prove irritating or even be toxic to the skin. Aromatherapy is most effective when it works on the mind and body simultaneously. The essential oils are added to the bath, massaged into the skin, inhaled directly or diffused to scent an entire room, used as a compress, salves, aphrodisiacs, medicated ghees, and patches, for hair care, cooking, dental care, in incense, candles, soaps. Specific blends are used to balance the doshas through panchakarma, shirodhara, tarpana, rasayana, kaya kalpa, chakra therapy and to treat allergies, arthritis, common cold, herpes, infections, gastro-intestinal symptoms, constipation, hemorrhoids, candidiasis, liver disturbances, ulcers, disorders of the gall bladder, intestine, pancreas, endocrine glands, hair growth, etc. Lemon oil taken internally or sniffed, is good for diabetes, asthma, boils and varicose veins. Three drops of sweet marjoram, taken with a little jaggery, cure migraine and hangovers. Nausea and vomiting are immediately controlled by petitgren oil. The ittar Gill or Itr-e-khaki, sondhi mitti drawn from mud extract, heals stubborn wounds, thanks to its antiseptic properties. Heena is known for its heat inducing qualities and if used on quilts during winters, it is known to provide extra warmth. Amber Heena is used for prayers, clairvoyance, protection from disturbing influences, insomnia and stimulates the 3rd Chakra. Musk ittar is derived from the juice of a mixture of flowers and is used mostly in tantrik rites, as also by males who want to woo the opposite sex.

The documented use of **Sandalwood goes back 4000 years** and caravans from Bharata to Egypt, Greece and Rome were a familiar sight. Many temples were built from Sandalwood and the Egyptians used it in embalming. Bharata migrants to Polynesia took sandalwood plants with them and Hawaiian history extolls its use in paying off the debt to white settlers. This relaxing oil is useful to treat tension, depression and nervous exhaustion; applied to the forehead it instills a sense of calmness for meditation. Sandalwood oil lessens stress and can stop vomiting, while applying it on the chest and throat cures dry cough and even skin ailments.

In Ayurveda, Rose is known as "The Queen of Flowers," for its romantic and feminine properties, and is said to symbolize **pure love**. It ignites a desire for romance and love and may help dissolve blockages, disappointment and pain. Rose petals also have the ability to maintain healthy cholesterol levels and rosewater is mildly astringent which makes it a valuable lotion for inflamed and sore eyes. Rose (Gulab) ittar's aroma relieves depression, frigidity, nervous tension, headache, shock, palpitations, poor circulation, nausea, sedative, runny nose, blocked bronchial tubes, insomnia, fatigue and irritability. It is anti inflammatory, enhances immunity, helps restrain infections through their cleansing action, gives a feeling of well being and happiness, calms a nervous mind, and cures respiratory tract as well as digestive problems. It can be used as an aphrodisiac and for skin care. Pink Rose oil reduces anger, depression and melancholy by dramatically soothing and strengthening the heart. Gulab ittar dominates both the heart chakra and the 7th chakra and balances all doshas. This ittar is widely used in puja of Lord Ganesha.

Champaka, also known as Frangipani, is a species of Plumeria, particularly sacred to Lord Krishna and, along with Ashoka flowers, also adorns the hair of the Mother Goddess Lalitambika. The five petals of the champaka or frangipani flower represent five qualities necessary for psychological perfection: sincerity, faith, aspiration, devotion and surrender. Shiva loves champaka flowers so much that he can bestow his blessings to anyone who offers champaka flowers. Champa ittar begins with sweetly innocent top notes, then evolves into a rich, magnolia-like floral with hints of spice. Sandalwood base notes help to ground the sweetness, giving it a refined balance. Champa Ittar can be worn as a lovely perfume, and is also used for **meditation**. Nag Champa has a strong, fresh, floral fragrance interspersed with a green note, appreciated for decades as exceptional incense, for meditation, and for creating one's own sacred space.

Mogra/Jasmin blossoms produce a sweet intoxicating aroma that is stronger at night than during the day. Called "The King of Flowers," Jasmine symbolizes **innocence, purity and nobility**. Jassmin ittar is 'Divine', stimulates the energy of the 5th and the 6th Chakras and is used to worship Lord Shiva. It helps to reach the inner self and is therefore used during meditation, for fast, and for lasting peace with one's own self. While morning-blooming Jasmine invokes the essence of dawn, night-blooming Jasmine invokes the fragrances of a moonlit grove on a warm summer night. Its sweet, cool, floral scent has a soothing, calming, mood enhancing and invigorating effect. Unarguably an important sensual aphrodisiac, Jasmine, is a scent associated with romance and seduction; men are automatically attracted towards women who use this ittar. It is believed to cure blood pressure, blood flow, stress, hypertension, skin ailments and insomnia.

The Lotus is India's national flower and its fragrance is seen as a **spiritual elixir**. It helps in meditation by calming the mind; promoting peace, serenity and improving concentration, hence quickening spiritual evolvement. Additionally, lotus flower essence hastens recovery from illness by enhancing healing at every level of the human body, and by equilibrating emotional imbalances. White Lotus is the **most sacred** spiritual oil in the world, revered as God's favorite flower, and its essential oil is a powerful aid to meditation, working directly on the Crown Chakra. White and green Lotus ittars are subtle, earthy, flowery scents that helps us transcend our earthly bonds and experience our Divinity. Lotus essential oils are perhaps the most expensive due to extremely low yields from the flower.

From Bharata, essential oils spread throughout the Old World. Egyptian papyrus scrolls mention aromatherapy with the aid of perfumed oils and scented barks, **imported from Bharata**. The inscription on the pyramid of Cheops (4500 BC) states: *"Every morning each slave will be provided a cove of garlic by his master for health and strength during construction"*. Special oils were used for each god and goddess and different perfumes were used for morning, evening, meditation, love, and war. Egyptian royalty had special perfumes blended for them and Queen Hatshepsut (1490-1468 BC) promoted perfumes as well as the bold eye makeup. Since a physical body was important in the afterlife, mummification required sequential impregnation with different aromatic oils, resins etc, all of which sometimes required six months for the royalty. The wrappings of early mummies were transported back to England and France, soaked in alcohol, and used as a medicine to increase resistance against disease. Cleopatra is believed to have bewitched Mark Anthony through her knowledge of perfumes. Imhotep, the Egyptian god of medicine and healing, recommended fragrant oils for bathing, massage, and for embalming their dead nearly 6000 years ago. Clay tablets reveal that in Babylon, 57,000 pounds of frankincense was burned every year. **Greeks and Romans borrowed heavily from Bharata and Egypt** and marketed the first commercial perfume, a reproduction of the Egyptian recipe named kyphi, dated 1500 BC. Hippocates recommended a daily essential oil massage, much as in Ayurveda, along with aromatherapy, baths, as well as aromatic fumigations to rid Athens of the plague. The body of Jesus was immersed in myrrh and other essential oils in an effort to revive it.

It was well documented that **herbalists and perfumers were virtually immune to common maladies**. A band of thieves could rob the house of black plague victims after drinking vinegar mixed with herbs and spices which made them immune to contagion. Avicenna (1000 CE) translated Sanskrit texts regarding distillation, perfumes etc and the **secret was carried back to Europe during the Crusades**. By 1200 CE, Germany alone was distilling 47 different types of essential oils which remained the best available medicine until the early 1900s. During WWII, Dr. Jean Valnet treated war injuries with essential oils and his student Margarite Mallory used aromatic oils in massage and skin care in England. The modern era dawned in 1930 when the French chemist Rene Maurice Gattefosse coined the term aromatherapy for the therapeutic use of essential oils in a book published in 1937. He was fascinated by the benefits of lavender oil in healing his burned hand without leaving any scars. **French blending** divides oils into narcotic and stimulating, or fresh and erogenous, an **improvisation of Ayurveda**. Later, Madame Marguerite Maury elevated aromatherapy as a holistic practice. The American Aromatherapy Association was founded in 1987 but other discoveries followed in Russia and Italy. Henry David

Thoreaux remarked:

> *"If the day and night are such that you greet them with joy and life emits a fragrance like flowers and sweet scented herbs - that is your success. All nature is your congratulations."*

Aromatherapy is one of the fastest growing fields in alternative medicine but the term itself has been excessively abused as there is no legislation to control it. Most of the ready-made products labeled with the word "aromatherapy" are neither pure nor natural. **Artificial products are even harmful** while, at best, they provide only a fraction of the benefit of the natural product. Buyers seeking true aromatherapy products must look at the ingredient label to ensure that the product does not contain fragrance oils or impure (chemical) components. A general rule-of-thumb is to be wary of products that do not list their ingredients and those that do not boast of having pure essential oils. Nevertheless, this 'therapy' is widely used at home as well as massage parlors, clinics and hospitals around the world for a variety of applications such as: pain relief during labor or caused by the side effects of the chemotherapy in cancer patients, and rehabilitation of cardiac patients. In Japan, engineers are incorporating aroma systems into new buildings. In one such application, the scent of lavender and rosemary is pumped into the customer area to calm down the waiting customers, while the perfumes from lemon and eucalyptus are used in the bank teller counters to keep the staff alert.

Astrology and Ayurveda. Eternally fascinated by the uncertainty of the future, man has attempted to peep into it by various means. **Astrology is a significant branch of Ayurveda** which scientifically studies planetary movements and their effect on human constitutions and lives. Planets are important indicators of spiritual and materialistic tendencies because each planet is intrinsically related to specific body tissues and various planetary movements exert powerful influences on the mind, body and consciousness. While the Sun is linked to circulatory deficiencies, anemia and indigestion the Moon is linked to circulatory disorders and lunacy. Mars is related to blood and liver and can cause pitta disorders such as constipation, flatulence, blind piles, and skin eruptions. Mercury affects reasoning, nervous diseases, ulcers, acidity, blood pressure, restlessness, and irritation. Venus governs semen, prostate, testicles, ovaries, bronchial disorders, whooping cough, asthma, dyspepsia, sexual ailments, delirium, and obsessions. Saturn is related to neurosis, neuralgia, sciatica, rheumatism, excretory disorders, muscle wasting and emaciation. Jupiter is related to jaundice, biliousness, colic problems, palpitation, toothache and insomnia. In Bharata Astrology, the sun, Rahu and Ketu are nodal points exactly opposite to each other and are given the status of planets. *Rahu* can influence hyperacidity, burning sensations, brain Disorders, sexual excesses and drinking problems. *Ketu* is related to skin disorders, nervous debility, small pox, and urinary tract infections.

To counter these negative planetary influences, Ayurveda suggests the use of **multi-faceted herbs** that not only provide curative relief to various physical afflictions but are also endowed with the preventive power to combat planetary interference. Afflictions related to the Sun, Moon, Mars, Mercury, Venus, Saturn, Jupiter, Rahu and Ketu are to be treated, respectively, with: *Aegle marmelus, Cueumis satirus* or Cucumber (*Khirika*), *Hemidesmus indicum* (*Anantmool*), *Bacopa monierri* (*Brahmi*), *Hydrocotyle asiatica* (*Mandukparni*), *Nyetanthes arbortristis* (*Shefali*) or *Desmostachya bipinnata* (*Dhuva*), *Bacopa monierri* (*Brahmi*), *Withania somnifera* (*Aswagandha*). The properties of the herbs can be increased by taking them with gem tinctures, or wearing the corresponding gems.

Planetary influences can also be vitiated by **gems and stones** that carry energetic vibrations with healing properties. Colors are related to bodily tissues and their vibrations are used to balance the tridosha by appropriate gems and precious stones. Gems can be left overnight in water which is consumed the next day and may be purified by putting them in salt water for two days. If a gelatinous paper of one of the seven colors is wrapped around a jar of water and left in sun light for four hours, the water becomes infused with the vibrations of the color and will help when drunk. Red (ruby or red coral) has a heating effect, promotes red blood cell formation, maintains the color of the skin, energizes nervous tissue, relieves kapha and vata but over exposure may cause conjunctivitis and inflammation. Orange (yellow sapphire and topaz) is warming, gives strength and energy to the sex organs but also helps the spiritual leader to renounce the world. It relieves vata, kapha, congestion, and also maintains the luster of the skin. Yellow (yellow sapphire or topaz) stimulates understanding as well as intelligence and is related to the complete death of the ego. Green (emerald) calms the mind, brings energy to the heart chakra, soothes emotions, calms vata and kapha but aggravates pitta. Overuse of yellow and green may cause stones in the gall bladder. Blue (sapphire) is pure consciousness, calming, cooling, relieves pitta but may aggravate vata and kapha. Purple is cosmic consciousness, creates lightness in the body, opens perception, relieves pitta and kapha but its overuse may aggravate vata. Although gems and stones can minimize the impact of planetary afflictions, they should always be worn with care and on recommendation of an experienced astrologer who would have a number of possibilities to choose from. Wrong stones can aggravate an existing condition and even cause fresh problems so caution is advised. Gems are also used for internal cleansing and Rasayans but they have to be treated with complex procedures to render them safe and non-toxic. Gem tinctures can be made by soaking the gem in 50-100% alcohol for various period of time that can be used for as long as one month for the diamond tincture.

Aura Therapy

Every substance in the universe, living or dead, emits energy which forms a **unique radiation** pattern termed 'aura', much like a fingerprint. Artists and mystics have from ancient times seen and portrayed this effect all over the world. Each person's aura is thought to be made up of the radiation from all the cells and chemicals within the body that derive their power from the omnipresent, universal energy. The visible aura, much in evidence in all religious texts, is said to be an oval extending from a few centimeters to a meter around the body, sometimes more at the head. The light rays are associated with different organs of the body whose variations in shape, color and strength are a reflection of each individual's uniqueness. The auras of plants, animals, and minerals are said to interact with one another as part of a single living system.

In 1911 Kilner published one of the first western medical studies of the "Human Atmosphere" or Aura along with possible use in medical diagnosis and prognosis. Glass slides or "Kilner Screens", containing alcoholic solutions of variously colored dyes, including a blue dye called "dicyanin", were used as filters in "Kilner Goggles" which, together with lights, were able to perceive electromagnetic radiation outside the normal spectrum of visible light. Closest to the body is the ethereal double, followed successively outwards by the inner aura (dark blue, green or pink) generally not detectable, outer blue and outer gold. The colors signify various mental states and vary according to the state of mental and physical health. Kilner's work was taken up by Theosophists and incorporated into Arthur E. Powell's book "The Etheric Double". Pranayama, mantras (AUM), silence, gems and meditation increase the aura while hospitals, machines, medicines and drugs weaken it. Dark gems like amethyst and blue sapphire protect the aura while ruby, garnet and red coral energize it.

Aura therapists believe that **personality and emotions** too can be interpreted **from auras**. One with soft, fringed edges, for instance, is likely to indicate a person too susceptible to the influence of others. Firm but fluid boundaries would indicate openness but not vulnerability. A hard, distinct outline belongs to one who is defensive and insecure. Lots of red within the aura would indicate anger while a predominance of blue would stand for idealism. Aura therapists believe that they have the skills to locate imbalances in the energy **linked to the chakras**, and that these imbalances can cause psychological as well as physical problems. Dr. Neva Dell Hunter pioneered the practice of aura balancing in which the practitioner works directly with the energy fields around the physical body. Aura Patches from various manufacturers, to be attached to the left side of the body, above the waist, deliver specific energetic frequencies which allow the body to heal itself naturally without any pharmaceutical or chemical compounds. These consist of colored essences, sprays and chakra-balancing oils, minerals, crystals, flower extracts, and gems. The idea is to balance color and light by adding extra colors to improve a dull or depleted aura or using complimentary colors to offset one that is too strong. However, active participation of the patient is extremely crucial to gain awareness of their spiritual potential.

Laughter Therapy (Gelotology)

Laughter is caused when the epiglottis constricts the larynx, thereby causing respiratory upset. Laughter depends upon neural paths in the telencephalic and diencephalic centers linked to respiration. While Wilson considered that the mechanism was to be found in the region of the medial thalamus, hypothalamus, and subthalamus. Kelly and co-workers postulated that the tegmentum near the periaqueductal grey contains the integrating mechanism for emotional expression. Laughter is not limited to humans, tickle a baby chimpanzee and it will giggle just like a human infant because laughter originated millions of years ago in one of our common ancestors. Laughter is used as a signal for being part of a group, it signals acceptance and positive interactions with others. Laughter is sometimes seemingly contagious, and the laughter of one person can itself provoke laughter from others as a positive feedback. Humor is a universal language, a contagious emotion, and a natural diversion. It connects people and breaks down barriers.

Laughter is found to lower blood pressure, increase muscle flexion, boost immunity by increasing T-cells, Gamma-interferon, and B-cells, decrease asthmatic attacks, increase stamina, relieve arthritic pain, ensure good sleep and elevate mood. Laughter also triggers the **release of endorphins** and produces a general sense of well-being, strengthens the cardiovascular functions, reduces stress hormones, improves circulation, promotes blood oxygenation by stimulating the respiratory system. Since serotonin levels go up after laughter, it is an effective antidote for depression. As blood vessels dilate, blood pressure falls by 10-20 mm mercury after 10 minutes of laughter. Laughter is additictive and hospitals around the US are incorporating formal and informal laughter therapy programs into their therapeutic regimens. Laughter therapy is not recommended in patients with hernia, advanced piles, eye complications, angina pain, major surgery, pregnant woman, tuberculosis, chronic bronchitis and phlegmatic respiratory infections. Finally, even a normal person experiencing discomfort while laughing, must discontinue immediately and seek expert medical help.

Haasya Yoga is a method of group laughter based on asanas, stretching, breathing and simulated laughs, starting with deep breathing. In Bharata, **laughing clubs** are becoming as popular as Rotary Clubs in the United States where participants gather in the early morning for the sole purpose of laughing. Thousands of laughter club members have decreased incidences of cough and cold. Exercise induced laughter permits the individuals to increase their capacity to laugh more, be more self-confident and self-expressive. Positive qualities are cultivated, thereby removing negative emotions as jealousy, fear, guilt and anger. The laughter club is in effect a behavior modification institute that spontaneously raises spirits at no cost. The concept of a laughter bank, where people come up with creative ideas for different types of laughter, is to bring fullness into the atmosphere. The fun, frolic and childish attitude not only reduce inhibitions but also curtail tensions.

Magnetotherapy

Magnetotherapy, or magnotherapy, is based on the principle that the **earth is one big magnet** and that all our bodies are surrounded by magnetic waves emanating from the earth and other spatial bodies, including the sun and moon, which influences and supports life. In the Yogic tradition, it is imperative that one align the body in correct magnetic field for meditation, hatha yoga postures, pranayama, meditation and sleep. Disease is caused by an imbalance between various electro-magnetic forces present within our bodies. Therefore, strategic placement of magnets on specific parts of the body can cure chronic ailments that standard medicine might find difficult to control. Legend has it that Cleopatra always wore a small magnet on her forehead to maintain her youth and beauty and that man in love kept magnets to keep their beloveds attracted. Magnetotherapy involves the use of permanent, static magnetic fields on the assumption that subjecting certain parts of the body to such fields has beneficial health effects. Products include: magnetic bracelets and jewelry; magnetic straps for wrists, ankles, knees, and the back; shoe insoles; mattresses; magnetic blankets; and even water that has been "magnetized". These devices are generally considered safe in themselves and application is usually performed by the patient himself.

Some of the basic principles of magnotherapy include: the use of **mutually opposite polarities of the North and South Poles**. Two methods, Unipolar and Bipolar, are used - the use of only one pole helps if diagnosis and selection of pole is correctly made. The patient is made to sit or lie down on an insulating wooden chair or bed. While the shape or size of the magnet does not matter, for sensitive organs like the eyes, brain and heart, weak magnets are used for very short periods of time, while for chronic ailments, strong magnets are needed. Therapy is never given on a full stomach, pregnant women should opt out of it, and all metallic objects that absorb magnetic waves should be removed. In the treatment of skin diseases, a cloth should be placed between the magnet and the skin.

Magnetotherapy is considered pseudoscientific due to both physical and biological implausibility, as well as a lack of any established effect on health or healing. Perhaps the most commonly suggested mechanism is that magnets might improve blood flow in underlying tissues. Although hemoglobin, the blood protein that carries oxygen, is weakly dimagnetic and is repulsed by magnetic fields, the magnets used in the therapy are many orders of magnitude too weak to have any measurable effect on blood flow. A 2002 U.S. National Science Foundation report on public attitudes and understanding of science noted that magnet therapy is "not at all scientific". A 2003 Cochrane Review on the treatment of the carpal tunnel found no improvement in symptoms between placebo and control. Similarly, a 2008 systematic review on magnetotherapy found no evidence for pain relief, with the possible exception of osteoarthritis. Both reviews report that small sample sizes, inadequate randomization, and difficulty with allocation concealment, all of which tend to bias studies positively, limit the strength of any conclusions. The worldwide magnet therapy industry totals sales of over a billion dollars per year, including $300 million dollars per year in the United States alone. A number of vendors make unsupported claims about magnet therapy by using pseudoscientific and new-age language. However, the U.S. Food and Drug Administration prohibits marketing any magnet therapy product based on medical claims.

Musicotherapy

Music can be defined as *"…a kind of inarticulate, unfathomable, speech which leads us to the edge of the infinite and lets us for a moment gaze into that"*. Music therapy has a long history dating back to the seven **Vedic chakras** each one of which was linked to a note of the octave (chapter 10). In the Old Testament, King David's court used the harp to cure illness and Hippocrates used it extensively. In ancient Egypt, pain of childbirth was similarly reduced by music. In Bharata legends, Thyagaraja was believed to have sung back life into the dead. The strongly developed **harmonic system** of **the Western music** is diametrically opposite to the **melodic Bharata system**. Although melody was the sole component of early Western music in the Gregorian chants, Pope Gregory in the seventh century completely revised them into the present form. The fundamental and most important difference between Bharatiya and Westen systems of rhythm is, respectively, one of **multiplication and addition of the numbers two and three**. The highly developed tala, or rhythmic system, avoiding strict meter and combining beat divisions, has no parallel in Western music. On the other hand, the Bharata system has no exact counterpart of the tempered Western music, except for the keynote. Considering the divergence between the two, it is not possible to imagine one borrowing from the other. **Pythagoras introduced the Vedic octave to Greece** and he came to be called the *'discoverer of the octave'* by the succeeding white imperialists. Arabs too had no musical tradition to start with and Arab writer Jahiz at the Abbasid court mentions Bharata instruments; many Indian terms also entered the vocabulary of Arabic music. Bharata *traga tala* was transformed into Arabic *maqam iqa* as the former existed more than a thousand years before the latter was known.

Basically, a sound (*nada*) generates particular vibrations which affect the human body via the chakras (Figure 7). In the classical Bharata system, it usually takes the form of a *raga* which has four sources - folk songs, poetry, devotional songs of mystics, and compositions of classical musicians. The articulation, pitch, tone and specific arrangement of *swaras* **(notes) in a particular** *raga* **stimulate, alleviate, and cure various ailments**. Ragas are closely related to the time of the day, season and emotional status. The muscles and nerves of the affected parts go through alternate contraction and relaxation during impulses and the in-between intervals. This enables energy from the universal field to flow into the human field and affects the central nervous system as well. Also, beats in the music have a close relation with heart beats; those below the pulse rate calm and relax while those above it excite and rejuvenate. While ragas can cure tension, blood pressure, heart ailments, insomnia and other disorders, such therapy should be conducted either in the early morning, evening or late night, never in long sessions on an empty stomach, and ideally with regular short breaks in between.

In the west, a trained music therapist uses music and all of its facets—physical, emotional, mental, social, aesthetic, and spiritual—to help clients improve or maintain their health. In a session with a musical therapist, one would improvise, recreate, listen, or compose their own piece.

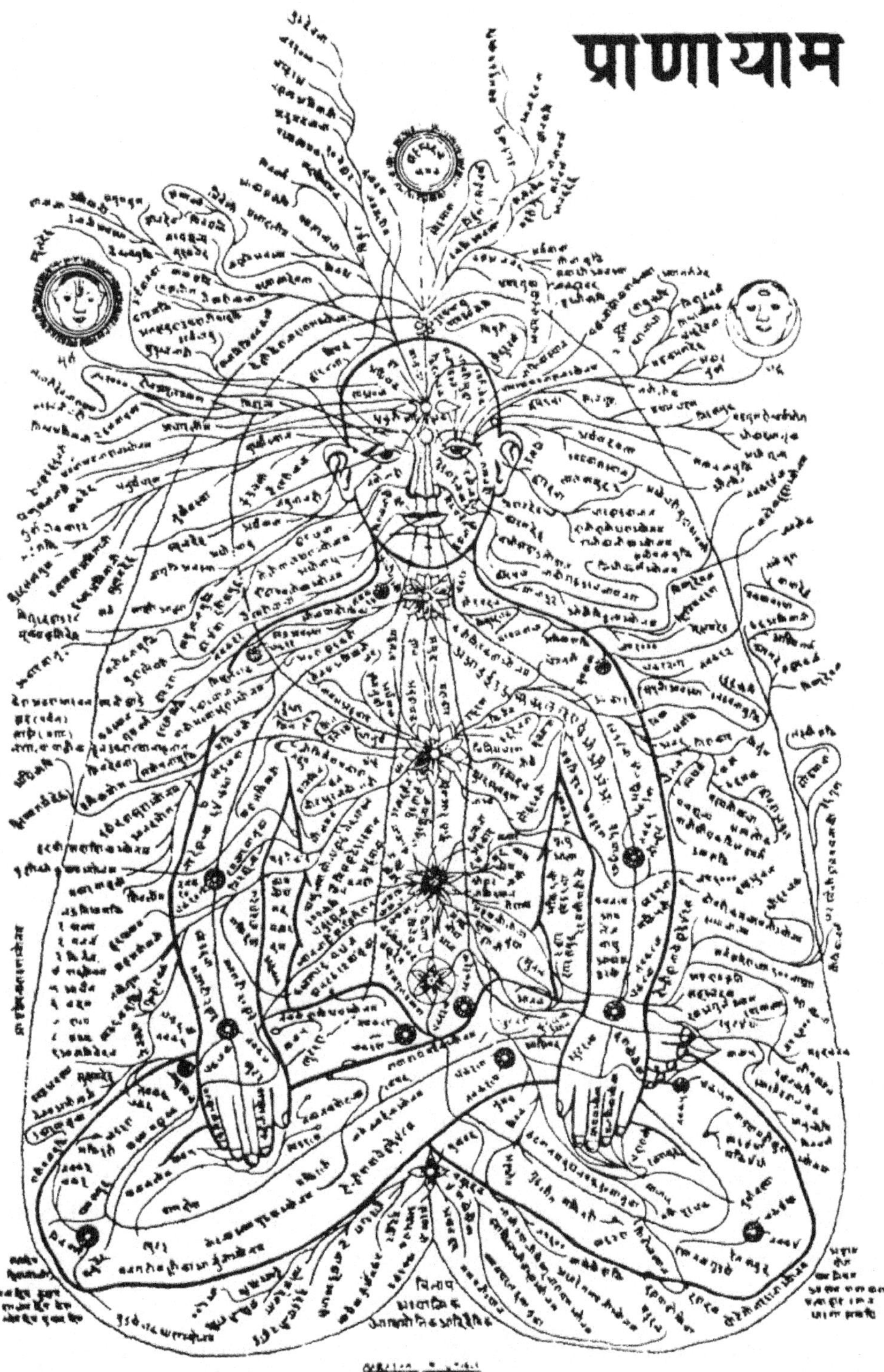

Figure 7. Vibrations and energy flow through nadis in the human body emanate as sound or Vac for speech and music. Pranayama and Yoga tune them back to their proper energy centers (source: an ancient manuscript, date and author unknown, from Wikipedia).

Each of these offers different benefits but all rely on the simple use of music to relay emotion between the therapist and the subject's inner emotional being. In improvisation, the subject would write entirely new lines of music based on their emotions, events, or situations which are brought up during a session. When composing, a client works with a therapist to create a piece of music where the therapist does the technical work if the client does not have sufficient knowledge of the musical theory. When simply listening, a therapist uses music to connect with the subject and urges it to reply to a piece with conversation about the emotions provoked by the song. According to Bruscia, the music may cause a client to recall a particular memory or even tell a therapist what words simply cannot convey, as music is the voice of the deepest most sincere emotion. Nayak et al. have shown that music therapy in stroke patients improves recovery as well as emotional and social deficits resulting from stroke. It decreases depression, improves mood, reduces anxiety, increases awareness, responsiveness, positive associations, mood, motivation, and the recovery of motor skills. Rhythmical auditory stimulation in a musical context, in combination with traditional gait therapy, improves the ability of stroke patients to walk. Music may reduce heart rate, respiratory rate, and blood pressure in patients with coronary heart disease and anxiety, according to a 2009 Cochrane review of 23 clinical trials.

In 1729 Richard Browne compiled the well-known *Medicina Musica*. Music therapy has existed in its current form in the United States since around 1944, when the first undergraduate degree program in the world was founded at Michigan State University, along with the first graduate degree program at the University of Kansas. The American Music Therapy Association (AMTA) was founded in 1998. To become board-certified in the United States, a music therapist must complete course work at an accredited ATMA program at a college or university, successfully complete a 1040 hour Music Therapy internship, and pass the Certifying Board examination. Current music therapists hold the designation, MT-BC, music therapist-board certified, given by the Certification Board of Music Therapists. A degree in music therapy requires proficiency in guitar, piano, voice, music theory, music history, reading music, improvisation, as well as varying levels of skill in assessment, documentation, and other counseling and health care skills depending on the focus of the particular university's program. Live music was used in hospitals after both of the World Wars, as part of the regime for some recovering soldiers. Clinical Music therapy in Britain was pioneered in the 60s and 70s by the French cellist Juliette Alvin, whose influence on British music therapy remains strong. Mary Priestley, one of Juliette Alvin's students, came to create Analytical Music Therapy which, together with the Nordoff-Robbins school of Music Therapy, form the two central forms of Music Therapy today.

Reiki

Reiki is believed to have begun in **Tibet** several thousand years ago where a system of sounds and symbols was developed to harness universal healing energies. Various healing systems, which crossed many different cultures, emerged from this single source which is now forgotten. Reiki (pronounced ray-key) is a Japanese word representing universal life energy which is all around us. It is derived from *rei*, meaning "free passage" or "transcendental spirit" and *ki*, meaning "vital life force energy" or " universal life energy". Dr. Mikao Usui, a Japanese Christian educator in Kyoto, Japan, rediscovered the root system in the mid to late 1800s. After Usui's death, Chujiro Hayashi, a former student of Usui, left the Usui Reiki Ryoho Gakkai and formed his own association. Hayashi simplified the Reiki teachings, stressed physical healing and used a rather codified and simpler set of Reiki techniques. Many Reiki teachers and practitioners aim to abide by these five principles, one translation of which is: **just for today: do not be angry, do not worry, be grateful, work with integrity, be kind to others**. *Karuna* is a Sanskrit word that is used in Hinduism, Tibetan Buddhism and Zen Buddhism, and translates as any kind of compassionate action. This system was established in the US by Katherin Milner, and is known today as "Tera Mai."

Reiki teachings claim that there is an inexhaustible, universal, "life force" that can be used to induce healing. Reiki **enhances the body's natural ability to heal itself**. Everyone can gain access to this energy by means of an attunement process carried out by a Reiki Master. Claims for such energy have no known theoretical or biophysical basis but Reiki is regarded as the most effective life energy with a maximum of vibration. Reiki involves the transfer of energy from the practitioner to the patient to enhance the body's natural ability to heal itself through the **balancing of chakra** energy. It is a holistic, natural, hands-on energy healing system that all at once touches body, mind, and spirit. Recipients decide subconsciously just how much of the Reiki energy is to be taken in. Those who use Reiki regularly often find they are more joyful, lively and their own in-built energy is enhanced-almost as if their batteries had been fully charged. Existing conflicts within the person are broken down and there is a greater vitality, leading to relaxation and a stimulation of the body. As this improvement progresses, the natural processes of renewal, and removal of toxins, are enhanced and rendered more effective, ultimately opening up more of the body to the life energy. Reiki is useful in treating serious illnesses as well as sports injuries, cuts, burns, internal diseases, emotional disorders, stress-related illnesses, skin diseases, and immunity.

The Reiki master acts as a channel and a link with God to release the healing power. An initiation is not absolutely essential but it conveys a greater capacity for using Reiki energy with no associated tiredness, and provides a protective mechanism against any negative manifestations. The therapist first makes a body-scan of the seven chakras to determine individual needs. Providing holistic, positive energy from the therapist to the client, without any side effects, it can be delivered independently or with other medical treatments. The reiki recipient should give up anger, honor parents, teachers and elders, earn living honestly, and show kindness to all living beings. Before the reiki session, the master should remove his/her own jewelry, wash hands, invoke higher powers, smooth the aura of the recipient, and finally give an energy stroke from the pelvis to the crown above the middle body. He then transfers reiki energy to the recipient in 17 positions that require 90 minutes. Special positions are used for diabetes, joints, multiple sclerosis, sciatica, heart attack. In the First degree stage, the subject gets attuned, as the universal energy activates the body, for approximately four hours over several days. After attunement, information is given on four levels of energy - physical, mental, emotional and spiritual. This stage provides deep relaxation, detoxification, receptiveness to universal life force and vibrations, as one opens up to a higher level of universal resonance. In the second degree stage, symbols are introduced to unlock the chakras. This treatment can be given at distance (no contact necessary) and requires 20 minutes. In the third degree stage, the subject is taught the intricate process of passing on the reiki energy and ways of enhancing personal growth and transformation.

Tibetan-Tantric Reiki uses 11 symbols of power four of which are called "Tibetan symbols," and the other seven are called "Tantric symbols." The Tantric symbols apparently come from the teachings of Shakyamuni Buddha, called Padmasambhava (Guru Rinpoche), who introduced Buddhism, to Tibet. The symbols fill the recipient with vital force and raise the Kundalini by activating the chakras. Each sacred symbol holds energy, represents a truth, and can be used to invoke its meaning to enhance the flow of the Universal Energy. They are like keys that open doors to higher levels of awareness through energies, chakras, mantras, and power. The use of these symbols is said to cure even cancer and AIDS.

What makes Reiki unique is that it **incorporates elements of just about every other alternative healing practice**: spiritual healing, aura, crystals, chakra balancing, meditation, aromatherapy, naturopathy, and homeopathy. The major and minor chakras can be opened harmoniously with Reiki, always balanced from the extremities to the center, followed by smoothing out of the aura. Rock crystal, rose quartz and amethyst are used, related to the 2nd, 4th and 6th chakras, respectively. Helpful aromatic oils include clary sage, patchouli, lavender, lemon verbena, and sandalwood. They are mixed 1:20 with sweet almond oil and applied with middle and index fingers in anticlockwise, circular, movements towards the center of the chakra. Two people can practice it for enhancement of relationship while several people can use it for group consciousness. Reiki softens the effects of allopathic drugs, enhances the effect of homeopathic drugs, and supports phytotherapy. Reiki is never used during anesthesia and caution is advised with pain killers, anticoagulants and cardiac stimulants. Reiki can be performed with plants, pets and animals as well. An animal knows when it needs reiki and for how long. Your pet will take the position for maximum effect and go away when it no longer needs it. Some practioners use it with horses and cats. Reiki can be used to treat leaves, seeds, roots and water for plants. If you perform reiki with a tree you will feel its calm and power, you give it reiki and the tree takes you in its aura. Trees can be good advisors if they trust you, reveal images or other impressions.

In March 2009, the Committee on Doctrine of the United States Conference of **Catholic Bishops** issued a decree (*Guidelines for Evaluating Reiki as an Alternative Therapy*) **halting the practice of Reiki** by Catholics, including Reiki therapies used in some Catholic retreat centers and hospitals: "*since Reiki therapy is not compatible with either Christian teaching or scientific evidence, it would be inappropriate for Catholic institutions, such as Catholic health care facilities and retreat centers, or persons.*"

13.

Prevention is Better than Cure

Diet and Nutritional science

Ayurveda works on the principle that prevention is better than cure. Its basic preamble is to replace bad with good to equilibrate the natural balance. *You are what you eat* is usually credited to Aesop in the West, but in Ayurveda the regulation of diet has always had great importance because it considers human body as the product of food which influences an individual's mental and spiritual development, as well as his temperament. Food material is just alien when we ingest it, to be transformed by the Agni into rasa but when Agni doesn't work properly, toxins are produced whose accumulation reduces immunity. The paramount importance of diet was underlined by both Charaka as **Prakrititah Ahita Tama Ahara** which mentions 19 types of *Viruddha ahara*, and by Sushruta under the caption of **Ekanta Ahita Ahara** which mentions 10 types of **viruddha ahara**. Ayurvedic concepts of *ahara* and *vihara* are concerned with diet and lifestyle to prevent diease so **ausadhi** (medicine) doesn't have to be brought in. The basic therapeutic approach is, '*that alone is the right treatment which makes for health and he alone is the best doctor who frees one from disease*'. All food is composed of the five elements, six tastes, and twenty attributes. To alleviate doshas, sesame oil is used for Vata and Kapha, honey for Kapha and Vata, and ghee for Pitta and Vata; *amlaki* is the best herb to preserve youth. All sweet taste, except honey, aggravates Kapha; sour, except amlaki and pomegranate, aggravates Pitta; bitter and pungent, except garlic and long pepper, aggravate Vata. The utility of food is determined by eight factors: nature, cooking, combination, quantity, habitat (climate), time of consumption, dietary rules, and the condition of the person.

Food is transformed first into chyle or rasa and then into the dhatus so lack of nutrients in food, or its improper transformation, leads to a variety of diseases. In contrast to the western notions where food just consists of protein, fat, carbohydrates, vitamins and minerals, ahara is concerned with the effect of food on the gunas to balance the doshas. Complete nutrition requires that all six tastes be available in our daily diet because all six tastes contain various proportions of the five bhutas. Food high in one bhuta increases the dosha which represents that bhuta and the ensuing imbalance produces ama.   Because jala and prithvi predominate in the body, sweet taste is required for strengthening them. Sweet food will thus increase kapha and decrease akash and vayu, or vata dosha. Food high in Agni increases pitta and decreases kapha. Body has the capacity to generate the vitamins it needs so external vitamins in excess may produce hypervitaminosis.

A strong appetite called **deepan,** which stems from good digestion or **pachan,** signals that the digestive system is ready for new food intake; do not burden the digestive system by eating when not hungry, do not eat to full capacity, avoid drinking cold liquids with meals, eat the main meal at noon in a calm atmosphere, avoid snacks between meals, fast once every one or two weeks, and avoid oily or fried foods. A weak or variable appetite needs rekindling of Agni by ginger tea and liquid diet until hunger returns. Appearance of acidity, gas, bloating and nausea, as well as sour or metallic taste on the tongue, indicate a sluggish digestion because ama is being produced. Improper elimination in the form of loose bowels, constipation, hard or sticky stool, all indicate ama production due to fermentation in the colon. Eat only small amounts of easily digestible food to restore good elimination or *anuloman*, the first thing in the morning.

Fresh foods, which are naturally sweet, not only blend all six tastes but also nourish as they are easy to digest and improve the sattvic quality. The most effective way to enhance sattva is meditation which permits us to transcend the daily routine and connect with the paramatma so we become sensitive to the needs of our bodies. Sattvic foods include fresh milk, ghee, butter, honey, fresh fruits, most vegetables, grains, basmati rice, whole wheat, oats, mung dal, nuts. Rajasic foods include onion, garlic, hot pepper, tomato, radish, chili, corn, spices, egg, fish, poultry, fried foods, spicy foods, colas, sodas. Tamasic foods inlcude red meat, alcohol, mushrooms, fried and fermented foods, cheese, dry milk all of whch require much energy for digestion. Meat may also have some side effects as killing triggers fear and anger in the animal leading to the release of adrenalin and other stress hormones. Meat will aggravate pitta and tax Agni for digestion; it will also increase rajas and tamas and reduce sattva. Modern research has shown that red meat eaters are prone to heart disease, cancer and degenerative disorders. Refrigerated and frozen foods no longer retain the sattvic quality and develop a kaphic nature; all food left overnight is called **paryushit** or lifeless food by Ayurveda and it is rich in tamas. No more than eight hours should elapse between food preparation and consumption. Chemical preservatives have an effect similar to freezing. Raw foods increase vata and reduce kapha so Ayurveda asserts that all food be cooked to increase Agni in the pitta zone of the body. Fermented foods, such as vinegar, alcohol, soy sauce, yogurt, cheese, yeasted breads, pickles, ketchup, are considered paryushit as they disturb the sweet and sour phases of the prapka digestion. Refined foods remove the fibrous covering which is essential for peristalsis leading to constipation and acceleration of vata. As Agni does not have enough time to metabolize them, they promote dhatu degeneration. Refined sugar passes undigested through rasa and rakta metabolism, immediately overloading the liver, pancreas, and other organs of the pitta zone. Sugar fermentation increases acidity which consumes minerals and other nutrients. The over consumption of sweets and chocolate depletes calcium in bones, one of the seats of vata, and has been directly related to tooth decay. Fried foods tax the ability of Agni to metabolize it, produce acidity in the stomach, and tamas in the mind. Additives, colorings and flavorings are indigestible, deplete Agni, and poison the body. Whereas a little bit of salt and sugar increase rasa metabolism and pacify vata, in excess they have a toxic effect, aggravate kapha, and desequilibrate the rajas-tamas balance. In moderate amounts, hot, spicy foods increase pitta secretions and digestion but in excess (pizza, Mexican foods, barbecue sauces, pickles, and mustard) they create indigestion and increase rajas. Carbonation vitiates vata and produces hyperactivity in the gastrointestinal tract which impedes absorption and promotes rajas. Allergies are caused by the inability of the body to digest particular foods; refrigeration of milk, and drinking it cold, greatly increases its kaphic influence and the ability to digest it; homogenization of milk augments vata.

People generally prefer food which balances their primary dosha. For example, kapha people shun rich, oily, cold and sweet foods as well as dairy products, going instead for warm pungent, spicy foods. Kapha people should eat food rich in vata i.e., foods that are light, dry and sharp, bitter, pungent and astringent. In contrast vata people choose foods that are rich in cream, oils, butter, ghee, dairy products, bananas, wheat, rice barley and corn to counteract vata's drying effect. Pitta people, because of a strong digestive Agni, eat large meals, sweet, milk, butter, ghee, most fruits, rice, barley, bitter and astringent foods, cool foods and drinks. Pitta people should avoid sour, pungent or salty foods. Vihara depends upon the ability to know what is good for us i.e. to have a sattvic mind. Aerobics improves cardiovascular function, oxygenation, mamsa and meda dhatus. Whereas kapha vikruti needs intense exercise, pitta vikruti can handle only moderate amounts; vata should exercise less than kapha or pitta as too much exercise aggravates vata. *Vyayama* means gaining energy by exercise through Surya namaskar, asanas, pranayama and meditation, in that order. Exercising the internal organs of the chest and abdomen removes ama and improves the movement of nutrients to the dhatus. Besides alternate nostril breathing, dinacharya should include salabhasana, pawan muktasana, bhujangasana and uddiyana bandha.

Vata reduction: Recommended food includes wheat bread, basmati rice, mung beans/dal, sweet potatoes, carrots, parsley, lemon, lime, grapes, strawberries, cherries, pineapple, plums, pumpkin, papaya, mangoes, dates, figs, avocados, radish, cooked onion, asparagus, red beet, almonds, walnuts, pine nuts; sesame oil is best but olive, almond, sunflower oils can be used also. In moderate quantities, vatas can consume corn, buckwheat, millet, rye, barley, chick peas, lentils, potatoes, cauliflower, celery, spinach, cabbage, broccoli, leafy salads, tomatoes, mushrooms, apples, pears, melons, chili, cayenne pepper, beef, lamb, rabbit, game, ice cream, eggplant, green beans, fresh peas, radish, okra, peppers, cucumber, anise, turmeric, basil, coriander, cinnamon, ginger, saffron, ajwain, sea salt. Vata people should avoid bread made with yeasts, most legumes, dry grains, soybeans, dried fruits, raw onion, pork, lard, refined sugar and chocolate. To reduce vata, consume warm food and drinks, oily foods, sweet, sour or salty foods. Massage every day with sesame and essential oils along with meat broth enemas. Avoid dark colors, fasting, dry foods, pungent, bitter or astringent foods, cold wind, dampness, excess travel, television, radio, movies, excess talk and thinking. Do non-exhaustive and non-vigorous exercise (swimming, walking). Keep warm in cold climate or live in a warm climate. Ama accumulated due to Vata can be burned by ginger, black pepper, fennel and calamus. Vata prakriti people should practice Sukhasana, Siddhasana and Padmasana, Vajrasana and Svastikasana and right nostril breathing (inhale right, exhale left) for 10-15 minutes every day. Use yellow, orange and red for meditation and wear, jade, peridot, topaz, citrine and gold. Daily, self administered, abhyanga massage in early morning or late afternoon is best, using warm, cured sesame oil. Avoid cold, windy conditions, too much stress, exercise and travel as well as foods that are cold, dry, rough and hard. Perform pranayama, meditation, and yoga. Dry nasal passages can be improved by applying some ghee or warm sesame oil into the nose several times a day.

Pitta reduction: Eat wheat, mung beans, cauliflower, alfalfa sprouts, celery, apples, sweet grapes, milk, cream, buttermilk, butter, ghee, coco nut, sunflower, soy, coriander, sucrose. In moderate quantities, pittas can comsume rice, oats, chickpeas, tofu, soybeans corn, buckwheat, rye, brown rice, lentils, millet, boiled onions, carrots, red beets, spinach, sweet potatoes, radish, avocado, lemons, lime, grapefruit, sour oranges, apricots, peach, bananas, coconut, sunflower, soy, cottage cheese, fowl, turkey, rabbit, basil, fennel, ginger, nutmeg, cloves, asafetida, raw sugar, apple syrup, candied sugar, and honey. Avoid raw onion, peanuts, pork, lamb, beef, shellfish, cayenne pepper, black pepper, garlic, refined sugar. To reduce Pitta, use cool foods, predominantly bitter and astringent along with herbs like katuka and barberry; boil one or two inches of grated ginger until one cup of water is reduced to ¾ and drink it around 10 PM. Next day eat only kichri. Have flowers around the house, take flower baths, and bathe in moonlight. Massage the scalp with coconut oil. Competitive team sports should also be practiced. Silver, sapphire, aquamarine, azurite can be worn on the right side of the body while blue and green should be used for meditation. Pitta prakriti people should practice Dhanurasana, Bhujangasana, Matsayasana, Sarvangasana and Halasana along with Shithali inhalation and Sitkari exhalation.

Kapha reduction: Kapha people should consume basmati, corn, rye, millet, barley, tofu, celery, cabbage, carrot, apples, pears, mustard oil, corn oil or sunflower oil, milk, buttermilk, turkey, chicken, rabbit, chili, cayenne, black pepper, garlic, ginger, cloves, cardamom, turmeric, cinnamon, honey, fresh vegetable juice from asparagus, beet green, bitter melons, broccoli, cabbage, carrots, cauliflower, kale and leafy greens. In moderate quantities they can also use brown rice, oats, chick peas, soybeans, potatoes, peppers, cauliflower, fresh peas, mushrooms, spinach, radish, leafy salads, onions, tomatoes, eggplant, okra, zucchini, sweet potatoes, cucumbers, dried fruits, dates, plums, lemon, lime, pineapple, oranges, melons, cherries, figs, mangoes, strawberries, raspberries, sesame, coconut, almond, cashews, walnuts, pine nuts, pistachios, and margarine. Avoid, white rice, wheat, bananas, peanuts, olives, pork, beef, lamb, refined salt, refined sugar, raw sugar, and maple syrup. To reduce Kapha, fast once a week for 24 hours and eat pungent, bitter and astringent foods. During fast, certain herbs such as ginger, black pepper, cayenne and curry, all of which are hot and spicy, may be used to neutralize the toxins. Fast rekindles Agni and since there is no food to digest, Agni burns away the toxins. Frequent, physical and mental exercise, and sexual, intercourse are recommended. Best colors are yellow, brown and red, and best stones are yellow topaz, corral and diamond. Use copper and iron on the body and take regular baths and saunas. Kapha prakriti people can benefit from Paschimotansana along with Ujjayi pranayama and Neti.

Rasayana therapy (use of immunomodulators and rejuvenation medicines) deals with the promotion of strength, vitality, memory, intelligence, immunity against the disease, youthfulness, luster, complexion, and optimum regeneration of the body and senses. Rasayana oils for vata, pitta, kapha are: sandalwood, aloe vera, and jasmine, respectively. Rasayana therapy is best after Panchakarma as it uses very refined and concentrated herbal and mineral formulae. Ashwagandha pacifies vata, brahmi and manjista pacify pitta, ginger and pippali improve digestion and pacify kapha, amalaki increases sattva. Substances with rejuvenating effects include: *Terminalia chebula, Terminalia belliric, Asparagus racemosus, Hydrocotyle asiatica, Glycyrrhiza glabra, Evolvulus alsinoidesm*, shilajit, detoxified metals, oxides from gold, silver, iron, mercury, pearls, diamonds, rubies, and more. More details on Rasayanas have been provided in chapter 15.

Dinacharya

In order to keep the tridoshas in a state of healthy equilibrium for proper digestion and metabolism, Ayurveda prescribes for each individual a specific daily routine (*dina* – day and *acharya* – behavior).

- Sleep before 10 PM and wake up at sunrise to synchronize biological clocks. Drink a glass of luke-warm water to flush out all toxins accumulated overnight in the body. Sleep no more than 6-8 hours. Gazing at the early morning sun or a candle is good for vision.

- Never suppress the natural urges like hunger, thirst, sleep, sneezing, yawning, vomiting, flatus and ejaculation, to avoid discomfort and even disease. Defecation once or twice daily is the best, though preferably not immediately after a meal, but urination then is wise. Examine the eliminations each morning and if poor digestion is noticed, go on a fast to correct the system before disease sets in.

- Thorough washing of the limbs, face, mouth, eyes, tongue, teeth and nose purifies the body's sense organs, occasional gargling with salt water, containing a pinch of turmeric, keeps gums, mouth and throat healthy. More advanced procedures include *jalaneti* for unhindered flow of prana, to temper cold, hay fever, headaches and migraines. *Jaladhauti* consists of drinking a glass of warm and slightly salted water and vomiting it out after 10 minutes. Keep hair trimmed and nails filed. Make an inhalation oil consisting of a mixture of 50 ml eucalyptus, 25 ml anise, 25 ml citronella, 25 ml clove, 50 g menthol crystals and 25 g camphor, shake well, store in a dark bottle, and allow to ripen for 15 days by shaking it daily. This mixture is put on burning soft coals or wood and inhaled.

- Regular exercise increases the body's stamina and resistance to disease by facilitating the immune system, clearing all channels, promoting circulation and waste disposal, and destroying fat. Depending upon the age and body type, kaphas can go for heavy exercises, pittas should do it in moderation while vatas should perform yoga and not aerobics. Never exert more than one half your capacity, during illness, just after a meal, and without rhythmic breathing. Meditation disciplines mind, controls desire, removes stress and anxiety. Recommended yoga postures are vata: lotus, vajrasana, siddhasana, alternate nostril breathing, surya bhedan pranayama; pitta: halasana, shoulder stand, shitali pranayama; kapha: paschimottan asana; neti and agnisara.

- A regular self-massage for 30 min with herbal oils, ghee or sesame oil is usually adequate but needs to be supplemented with professional attention, occasionally.

- Clothing should be light and airy, made of natural fiber like cotton, wool, linen or silk. Always use your own, and never somebody else's clothes, except that of a saint. Since energy is brought into the body through the crown of the head and exits from the soles of the feet, energy usually collects in the footwear. So avoid wearing someone else's footwear, try not to take shoes into the house and walk barefoot whenever possible; wooden sandals are more healthy than animal skin or rubber shoes.

- Eat in silence, be aware of food, fast once a week, brush teeth after meals, wash hands before and after meals, breakfast 8-10 AM, last meal 8 PM. Start out by eating something sweet to reduce pitta, followed by something sour and salty to stimulate digestion. A tea spoon full of grated ginger with a pinch of salt is a good appetizer. Lassi with ginger or cumin, or one tea spoon of ghee, helps digestion. A glass of warm milk at bedtime nourishes the body and calms the mind. Water taken before or after meals adversely affects digestion. Water should be stored in a copper vessel or with some copper coins in another container; this is good for liver and spleen. Excess of cold drinks reduce resistance and increase mucus.

- Sound sleep for 6 to 8 hours is essential as it promotes growth and relaxes, head pointing east feet west. Retire early on an empty stomach; while sleeping on the right side is the most relaxing, that on the left improves digestion and increases interest in food, sleep and sex. Sleeping on the back indirectly, and on the stomach directly, encourages disease. The ideal form of sleep is ***yoganidra*** – a state of complete physical inertness with retention of mental alertness and awareness. Washing hands, feet and face, just before retiring, improves sleep. Do not close all windows, and do not bring pets into your bedroom. A few relaxing yoga exercises and some meditation are recommended before retiring to bed.

- Often an extension of the owner's personalities, pets should ideally be chosen so as to have a therapeutic effect on the dosha imbalances. Vatas get along famously with dogs, while cat is the favorite for Pittas; Kaphas prefer birds.

- Choosing the right partner who will stimulate and inspire is very important. Upanishads compare the sexual act to a ritual and sacrament, and a progeny is the duty of every individual. Sex can be enjoyed at will during the winter season (December - March), every fourth day in spring (March - June) and autumn (September - December), and every fifteen days in the summer (June – September). A warm bath is recommended after the intercourse along with milk heated with raw cashews and raw sugar to promote strength and maintain sexual energy. Sex immediately after meals is injurious as is too much masturbation. Oral and anal sex cause vata degeneration.

- Since work consumes at least one-third of our lives, the nature of work should match well with prakriti. Vata people love work that requires sudden bursts of intense energy, need adequate rest, especially in the afternoons, and should avoid places where the air is exceptionally cool or dry. Pitta people are very practical, making good administrators but not original thinkers. Kapha stability and balance makes them great administrators as they make conscious effort to bring in change or variety to their otherwise staid and routine lives.

Ritucharya

As prakriti denotes both body constitution and nature, it is only to be expected that changing of the seasons will influence bhutas and thereby the doshas. Ayurveda divides the year into **six _ritus_** (seasons) – _varsha (monsoon), sharada (autumn), hemanta (winter), shishira (late winter), girshma (summer) and vasanta (spring)_. Cold, dry weather enhances vata, hot humid climate increases pitta, while cold, wet weather aggravates kapha. To avoid such imbalance, Ayurveda prescribes a seasonal routine to preserve the dosha balance by a unique _ahar_ (diet), _vihara_ (mode of living) and _karya_ (routine living). During spring, gargle with a warm saline solution in the morning to clear mucus from the nose and throat, and take a warm shower to dilate the shrotas to expel kapha. Apply ghee inside the nostrils against allergens and pollen. In the summer, Agni gains strength so eat light food with little spicing, take a nap in the afternoon to increase kapha, and eat a vata-reducing diet. In the autumn, vata's drying influence increases so oleation is recommended along with an appropriate diet to pacify both vata and pitta. Winter cold necessitates internal and external oleation, rasayanas, basti and nasya. The diet should be sweet and highly seasoned during the winter, early spring, and late fall, with plenty of oils, fats, wine, salty and sour food, and alcoholic drinks. During the spring, the diet should be mainly tangy and bitter while in the summer it should be sweet and highly flavored and devoid of alcoholic beverages. Cooked food is always preferred over raw.

Self Care at Home

Some **80% of the diseases are self limiting** and body can take care on its own. The most precious possession of an individual is the own, spiritual self. Negative energies are the root cause of ailments so spiritual therapies redirect the energies back on the right track. It is important that one should attempt to **root out all negative thoughts** from the mind and to concentrate on only the positive ones. The negative thought patterns which cause ailments are **anger, criticism, resentment** and guilt. It is utterly impossible to maintain a healthy body under such distressed condition. For instance, criticism over long periods will often lead to disease such as arthritis. Anger turns into constituents that boil and burn, and in the long run infect the body leading to heart ailments. Resentment eats into the system and ultimately leads to tumor and cancer. Guilt always seeks punishment and leads to all sorts of pain. **Hatred is the most severely damaging** mental activity; it poisons the body and mind and its effects are almost permanent. Next to hate, worry is just about the worst form of self-destructive mental activity. A person who exercises, meditates and thinks positively, is telling his body that he/she wants to stay healthy throughout life. Metaphysical causation transforms thoughts and words into actual physical parameters. For example, a stiff neck could easily be indicative of inflexibility in a person to listen to the other side of an argument. In Buddhist tradition, humility was to be gained by 100,000 prostrations.

To release tension, inhale to full capacity, retain for about 10 seconds, and exhale forcefully in three steps as if whistling by curving the lips. To produce heat in the body, close one nostril and inhale through the other to full capacity, close both nostrils, retain inside as long as possible, then exhale through the other nostril. To get over the feeling of hunger and thirst, make a sound with the throat while the mouth is closed. Gulp down the air thus produced inside the mouth as if drinking water. To get rid of tension, send prana energy to the tense part by becoming aware of the body; a massage will also help. Noise and pollution create acidity, obstructed breathing, and vitiation of the humors; asthma and chronic cough are directly related to the intake of prana so clear nasal passages with aromatic oils before going to bed and perform jalaneti upon rising.

Tarpana is based on the premiss that our thoughts are the most important factors in our well being. Tarapana is performed in a dimly lighted room, lit with candle and burning incense, along with the favorite essential oil in an aromatherapy lamp, or diffuser. Re-birthing breath, or connected breath, is used where inbreathing with the nose is followed by breathing out through the mouth to allow the exhalation to lead you to your own pace. Starting with the parents, each ancestor is called in return, visualized standing in front of you and receptive to anything you have to say. Tell them your feelings, look and see if you are willing to forgive, leave your feelings behind, and not carry it with you anymore. Thank them for the gift they have given to you: *"I have learned from this experience, I have grown, I thank you"*. Let your mind's eye offer to them their favorite food or drink. Visualize them taking it from your hand, consuming it and smiling. Hear them wishing you success in life, to find your own path, freeing you from any obligation so you can pursue your passion and your purpose. Accept this blessing and visualize them walking off into their own path, bless their path as they leave. Bring forth each of your ancestors and all others to free yourself. End your session by saying the deepest of all affirmations about yourself: *I am love, I am one with all things, I am peace, I am joy, I am prosperity, I am forgiveness, I am fulfillment etc. And so it is.*

14.

Contemporary Maladies and Management

AIDS. HIV virus attacks the CD34 cells that are causal to immunity via generation of antibodies to pathogens. In the Ayurvedic tradition, AIDS stems from depleted ojas due to excessive sex, drugs, poor diet, junk food, worry, insomnia, and the like. Both anti-pitta and anti-vata regimes should be followed along with a sattvic life style. Ojas should be increased by sesame seeds and oil, almonds, chick peas, milk, ghee, shilajit, ashwagandha, shatavari, gokshura, bala, kapikacchu, gotu kala, sarsaprilla, and Brhama rasayana. Diamond ash (hira bhasma) and mercury compound (Makardhwaj) are also beneficial, as are AUM and gems (yellow sapphire, yellow topaz, citrine, diamond and zircon). In contrast, AIDS therapy in the West is limited to products that inhibit viral replication and/or maturation in an effort to increase the CD34 cell count.

Allergy. The word allergy is derived from the Greek words "allos," meaning different or changed and "ergos," meaning work or action. Allergy is known in the western medicine only since 1900, defined as an exaggerated reaction by the immune system in response to contact with certain foreign substances. A complete description of allergy in Ayurveda can be traced under the title of "*Satmya*" (Charaka Sutra. 6/50): all those *Ahara* and *Vihara* which are having *Viruddha Guna* of a particular Dosha or Roga are considered as *Satmya* of that *Desha Roga*. *Satmya* is divided into 4 types: *Ritu Satmya, Auk Satmya, Desha Satmya,* and *Roga Satmya.* There are three main types of allergies: excessive dryness or vata allergy; inflamed sinuses or pitta allergies; and congestion or called kapha allergy. These stem from poor digestion and elimination, deterioration of the nervous system, physical and mental stress, decrease in the body's natural balancing and self-repair ability, all in relation to changing seasons. Accompanying signs include constipation, congestion, gas, diarrhea, headaches and skin rashes.

A specific diet regimen (Ahara and Vihara) is indicated to control allergy according to the season or *Ritu Sandhi* where a specific Dinacharya is to be followed for a period of about 14 days between two consecutive seasons. Herbs such as asafetida, ginseng, ashwagandha and shatavari are taken over a long period along with herbal combinations to increase absorption. Burdock root tea is the best blood-purifier for allergy, rash or acne, and is to be taken every night. Other blood purifiers include sandalwood, saffron, turmeric, calamus root powder, pomegranate juice, orange juice, and asparagus root. These may be combined with phlebotomy or taken on their own if the conditions and symptoms are mild. Anti-allergy herbs include: turmeric, guduchi, tulsi, *Picrorhiza kurroa*, *Tinospora Cordifolia*, Triphala, Mahalakshmivilasa rasa, Swansakuthar rasa, Swansakas chintamani rasa, Abhrakya bhasma hajarkuti, Talishadi churna, Siringadi churna, Sitopladi (dalchini, ilayachi, long, black pepper), Chyavanprasha, and Chittra haritki.

Other remedies consist of *Nasya* by Anu tail: for Vata and Kapha allergies, trikatu, basil, cloves, camphor, and coriander are used; to ease Kapha aggravation guduchi tablets may be taken along with basil, cloves, and camphor; for skin allergy use neem, Khadiraristam, Nimbasavam, Haridrakhandam, Agasthya rasayan; for allergy of the respiratory system use Agasthya rasayana, Nimbarajanyadi tablet, Spetilin Tablet, Septilin syrup, Kanchanar guggulu, Anu oil. For healthy resistance to all airborne allergens use Agasthya rasayana, Nimbarajanyadi tablet, Septilin tablet, Septilin syrup, Kanchanar guggulu, Anu oil, Cutis oil, and Haridra capsules. In Western medicine, allergy is generally treated with antihistamines and steroids to alleviate symptoms while desensitization to the etiologic agent is also possible in some cases.

Arthritis: Inflammation and degeneration cause arthritis and some 100 types are known, though the underlying factors remain unelucidated in allopathy. Ayurveda says that arthritis is caused primarily by an excess of ama vata, lack of Agni due to poor digestion, and a weakened colon that allows the toxins to reach the joints; pitta, and kapha types are also known. It is therefore important to stimulate Agni and to suppress the ama by hot, spicy foods and herbs, including galangal and cayenne. Haritaki, Amalaki and Bibbitaki are used to treat vata, pitta and Kapha types, respectively. Ruby, garnet or other "hot" gems set in gold are used for all three types of arthritis. Mahanarayana oil mixed with sesame oil (1:1) is applied to the painful areas, followed by, warm heat, yoga, bath, and mild exercise. Narayana oil is good for muscle and joint pain, lower body circulation, and reversing imbalances caused by aging. Avipattikar churna is good for rheumatism. Recommended yoga postures are: triangle, tree, forward bends, spinal twist, boat, bow, camel, cow, locust, chest-knee, mahamudra, and half bridge.

Herbs for arthritis include ashwagandha, ajistha, akarkara, haridra, turmeric, asafetida, garlic, ginger, licorice, guggul, Vatviduansa rasa, Rasaraja rasa, Vatchintamani rasa, Brahdabad chintamani, triphala gold pearl, mint, ephedra, golden seal, gentian, nirgundi, eucalyptus leaves, prasarini, quassia, coptis, scute, phellodendrom, aloe, guggul, Siberian ginseng, myrrh, *Apium*

Graveolens (Celery), *Moringa oleifera* (Horseradish), *Boswellia serrata* (Indian Frankincense) and yucca. One simbanada guggulu tablet (350 mg.) 3 times a day, and 1 chitrak-adhivati (200 mg) tablet twice a day are recommended. A quarter teaspoon of yogaraj guggulu, washed down with a little warm water 3 times a day, is also recommended. **Gout** is similar to arthritis where uric acid is deposited in the joints. Ayurveda calls it vatartaka or vata in the blood so the treatment aims to reduce vata and cleanse the blood. In the Western tradition, symptomatic medication includes anti inflammatory agents and steroids.

Cancer: Cancer is defined as uncontrolled proliferation of cells due to gene damage by certain chemicals and transformation by viruses. It seems that the seers of Ayurveda knew this fact **thousands of years ago.** Ancient Ayurvedic classics by Charaka and Sushruta also mention clinical features of cancer under the titles of *Apachi, Gulma, Granthi* (minor neoplasm), and *Arbuda* (major neoplasm), as inflammatory or non-inflammatory swellings. The decrease in Agni is inversely proportional to *arbuda* while *dhatwagni* (deranged metabolism) will result in excessive tissue growth. Sushruta described six stages in the pathogenesis of tumor: *Sanchaya* or localized neoplastic changes; *Prakopa* or transformation of primary growths into metastatic tumors; *Prasara* or metastasis; *Sthana samsraya* or complete metastasis with secondary growth; *Vyakti* or clinical signs and symptoms; *Bheda* where differentiation of growth occurs on the basis of histopathology. In the 8th century CE, Vagbhata composed two texts: *Ashtanga Hridaya* and *Ashtanga sangraha*, followed by Chakradatt by Chakrapani (10th century CE), the *Sarangadhara Samhita* by Sarangadhara (14th century CE), the *Bhavaprakasha Samhita* by Bhavamisra (15th century CE), the *Satmya Darpan Samhita* by Viswanath (16th century CE), the *Vaisajya Ratnabali* by Binoda Lala Sen Gupta (18th century CE), and the *Rasatarangini* by Sadananda Sharma (19th ccentury CE).

During the 7th century BC, **Atreya and Dhanwantari used herbal medicines to treat early stages of cancer,** and surgery in advanced cases. Many herbs used for the treatment of *arbuda* are bitter and immunostimulant but others include: red clover, burdock root, guggul, turmeric, saffron, chaparral, green tea (*Camelia sinensis*), cat's claw (*Uncaria tomentosa*), manjishta (*Rubia cordifolia*), periwinkle (*Vinca rosea*), shatavari (*Asapargus racemosus*), brahmi (*Bacopa monniera*), bullatacin (Andrographis paniculata), *Phyllanthus niruri/amarus, Piper longum*, podophyllin (*Podophyllum hexandrum*), *Tinospora cordifolia, Semecarpus anacardium*, triphala, and aswagandha. Because **Ayurveda views cancer as a psychic disorder,** due to an excess of *Apana*, a disruption in the aura can be repaired by gems such as the blue sapphire, diamond, ruby, garnet, red coral, emerald and peridot. Spiritual remedies include pranayama, meditation, and mantras like OM and RAM. Western treatments include surgery, irradiation, antimetabolites and antisteroids.

Circulatory System and Heart diseases: Whereas Western medicine considers brain as the ultimate center of control, Ayurveda believes that the heart is the seat of human consciousness or soul. Ayurveda mentions '*Hrudroga*' where the heart is defined as the organ responsible for controlling and monitoring emotions, as also for blood circulation. It is the seat of prana, ojas, and atman, the true or divine self, and of all of the main blood vessels. The **Vata is responsible for heartbeat and for the overall circulation** of the blood, Pitta for the metabolic enzymes in the heart, and Kapha for strength. Krimi type and Tridosha type of heart diseases have been described as well. The high death rate from heart disease in western countries stems from over emphasis on personal achievement that alienate the individual from family, friends and social interactions. The Western diet rich in sweet, salty and food fried in animal fats makes one prone to heart attacks, as do the sedentary and sluggish lifestyle, the lack of proper exercise, physical or emotional trauma, congenital or hereditary factors, suppressed emotions, excess strain and anxiety.

Recommended are low calorie vegetarian foods, oatmeal, corn apples, fresh fruit juice (orange or grapefruit), millet, and most fresh vegetables. Quit smoking, exercise regularly, remain calm and composed, laugh a lot, avoid coffee, tea and intoxicating drinks. Practice meditation 10 to 20 minutes twice a day along with shavasana. Mix garlic with butter milk and drink it twice daily. Dip fenugreek in water over night and chew in the morning on an empty stomach. Recommended herbs include: jaharmorha, nutmeg, Brahma Rasayana, saraswat powder, sarsaparilla, guggulu, cardamom, cinnamon, ashwagandha, sandalwood, saffron, Hawthorn Berries, myrrh, ginger. In particular, 1/2 teaspoon (500 milligrams to one gram) Arjuna 3 times a day with honey and warm water is highly recommended. Rudraksha can be used as a necklace of beads in front of the heart. **Ayurvedic herbal tea** is prepared by placing ½ tea spoon full of 1 part punarnava, 4 parts kutki, 3 parts gullvel sattva, 1/4 part shilajit in a cup of hot water taken twice a day after lunch and dinner.

Gold is good for the coronary artery and is said to reduce cholesterol so gold and copper water should be taken daily. Drinking rudraksha water is believed to reduce blood pressure and strengthen the heart. It is prepared by placing a rudraksha bead in water overnight and the water is drunk next morning; gold water is prepared similarly. Water purified by keeping it in a copper vessel overnight is good for heart as well. Gold, ruby and garnet stimulate and restore the heart while silver, jade, moon stone, emerald and pearl calm the heart. Yellow sapphire and yellow topaz tonify and strengthen the heart. For blood purification, make a powder containing 15 g each of kalongi, cress seeds, ajwain, basilica leaves, fenugreek, wormwood leaves, neem and atees. Swallow ½ tea spoons with water before going to bed for 15 consecutive days, twice a year.

A reading of 140/90 mm Hg or higher defines **Hypertension**, due primarily to a thickening of arterial walls so the heart has to do more work to pump blood. According to Ayurveda, hypertension is caused mainly due to accumulation of toxins in the blood and tissues, poor digestion or nutrition, imbalance of nervous system, and physical or mental stress due to disruption of natural biological rhythm. Salt (water and fire) favors hypertension and is commonly a pitta condition; however, also known are vata and kapha hypertension. Follow low salt and low fat diet, avoid alcohol and tobacco, walk for 30 minutes every day, practice some aerobics and yoga. The main herbs to reduce blood pressure include sarpagandha, Arjuna, punarnava (*Boerhavia diffusa*), rose extracts, and others. *Dhara* is beneficial in pacifying the mind and reducing blood pressure. Mix well ashwagandha 1 part, valerian 1 part, gotu kola 1 part, and take 1-3 grams of the powdered herbs either with warm water, or ghee. For Pitta hypertension use: aloe gel, barberry, katuka, rhubarb, senna, Brahma Rasayana, Saraswat powder, gotu kola and skullcap, in equal proportions. For vata Hypertension use: an entire crushed clove (with honey) once or twice a week, and nutmeg or saraswat powder in warm milk. For kapha hypertension use: cayenne, myrrh, garlic, motherwort and hawthorn berries, arjuna, trikatu, serpagandha ghana bati, arogyaavardhani, kanchanar gugul, ashwagandha, and hridyavasthi, but avoid licorice, **Hypotension** stems from the weakness of the digestive fire and treated with turmeric, cinnamon, ginger, cayenne, garlic, aconite, pippali and cardamom. **Epistaxis** (nose bleeding) is treated with sesame oil in the nose. **Hemorrhage** is primarily a pitta disorder, but other types exist as well, to be treated with a cold shower and herbs like aloe, majishta, saffron, alum, turmeric, Arjuna, ashok, and triphala. **Anemia** is a pitta disorder but other types also exist. Generally it is treated with red meat, bone soup, milk, black sesame seeds, iron, chyavan prash, turmeric ghee, aloe gel, amalaki, haritaki, saffron, shatavari, majishta, purnava, triphala ghee, raw sugar, and herbal wines (Draksha). Gems to wear include red coral, garnet and ruby. Allopathy uses a number of products for the symptomatic treatment of diseases related to the heart and circulation and surgery is practiced with these same goals in mind.

Diabetes Mellitus: The name is derived from Greek diabetes or *siphon*, and *mellitus* or sweet, due to insufficient production of insulin by the beta cells of the pancreas, an excess of glucagon, to be treated by diet and exogenous insulin. The Samhitas describe diabetes as *madhumeha* (honey urine), primarily a kapha disorder, due an excess of sweet (earth and water) and obesity. Avoid sweets, fats, eat bitter vegetables, quit smoking and alcohol, do some daily exercise like cycling, swimming, jogging etc along with Bhujanga asana, Salabha asana, and Dhanur asana. Rasayans to treat diabetes include a combination of: neem (*Azadirachta indica*), gurmar leaves (*Gymnema sylvestre*), karela (*Momordica charantia*), nayantatra (*Vinca rosea*), jambhul (*Eugenia jambolana*), sagar gota (*Ceasalpinia crista*), bel (*Aegle marmelos*), turmeric, katutikt, harsingar, Pramehagaja kesari, vangabhasma, aloe, shilajit and gurmar (*Gymnema sylvestre*).

Digestive System Dysfunctions: Proper management of the colon is causal to treating digestive disorders, related primarily to the root chakra, whose symptoms and treatments are dosha-dependent. While **diarrhea** results from lack of absorption of nutrients, constipation is the retention of waste material. Good spices for diarrhea include ginger, long pepper, saffron, coriander, cardamom and nutmeg, taken with buttermilk. **Constipation** can be treated with many herbs (asafetida, ginger, cardamom, fennel) triphala, and enema. An excess of gas and **colic** stem from ama accumulation due to high vata to be treated with herbs such as cardamom, fennel, ginger, peppermint, orange peel, bay leaves, ajwain, asafetida, valerian, nutmeg, chamomile, as well as formulae like Trikatu and Trisugandhi. **Hemorrhoids** are caused by varicosity of the veins around anus where diet should be modified according to the predominant dosha, along with the intake of the corresponding herbs. **Nausea** (vomiting) is a disorder of the stomach due to an excessive upward movement of udana vayu. Anti-emetic herbs include ginger, fennel, basil, nutmeg, cardamom, and cloves; cardamom and fennel in equal parts with honey will stop almost every kind of vomiting. **Hyperacidity** stems from aggravated pitta due to spicy, greasy, sweet or sour food and alcohol consumption. An anti-pitta diet (basmati rice, milk and ghee) is to be followed along with herbs like aloe, shatavari, amalaki, licorice, marshmallow, gentian, barberry, conch shell (shankha bhasma), asafoetida, trikatu, and herbal antacids. Also helpful are: pomegranate juice, one tea spoon full of licorice root powder and turmeric powder, three times a day in between meals; tea made out of one tea spoon full each of fennel, cumin and coriander, in two cups of water boiled down to one cup, is taken for two to three days. **Ulcers** are an inflammation of the mucosal lining of the stomach and stem from vitiated pitta; the treatment is the same as for hyperacidity. The **liver** is a pitta organ and many pitta disorders (infections and inflammations) originate there. Aloe gel is an excellent liver tonic, taken 2-3 times a day, while the best Ayurvedic herb for liver is Bhuyamalaki (*Phyllanthus niruri*) which can even cure Hepatitis B. An anti-pitta approach should be combined with raw vegetables, fruits, ghee along with herbs (coriander, fennel, cumin, turmeric, cyperus, mint, lemon and lime). **Hepatitis** (jaundice) is a viral disease but wrong diet and pitta aggravation can increase susceptibility to infection. The treatment is strongly anti-pitta: bitter herbs (katuka, barberry, nishot, guduchi, gotu kala, bhringaraj, chiretta, aloe gel) and formulations like Sudarshan powder. Gall stones or **cholecystitis** is caused mainly by congestion and obstruction in the flow of bile due to deranged pitta, to be treated with liver cleansing herbs and liver tonic.

The small intestine (*grahani*) is the seat of Agni whose dysfunction can give rise to constipation, diarrhea, gas, fatigue, low energy, problems of appetite, decreased resistance, and malabsorption syndrome. A buttermilk fast is followed by kichri and food containing pungent and astringent spices (ginger, asafetida, cinnamon, cumin, haritaki, cloves, cinnamon) that improve absorption, as well as combined formulations. **Anorexia** can be treated with ashwagandha, gotu kola, chyavan prasha and sesame oil massage. **Hiccups** can be alleviated with honey and castor oil, along with correct breathing and meditation. Internal bleeding is treated with warm milk containing saffron and turmeric powder.

Ear, Eyes, Nose and Throat: To alleviate pain, garlic oil, or onion juice with honey, can be introduced in the painful ear; for ringing sensation in the ear clove oil is used. To ease burning sensation, introduce rose water or fresh aloe vera gel into the afflicted eye. Toothache can be treated with clove oil applied to the affected tooth. **Cough, laryngitis and sore throat** stem from deranged kapha, pitta or vata   but dry cough is primarily a vata type disorder. Ayurveda describes cough as *Kaasa roga* due to deranged vata but other doshas contribute as well. Cough stems from internal infection and may be accompanied by low fever. Herbs recommended are: *Pelargonium sidoide*, bay berry (*Myriad nagy*), belleric (*Terminalia belerica*), betel (*Piper betel*), butea (*Monosperma aromaticum*), *Euphorbia hirta*, fenugreek (*Trigonella foenum graecum*), and henna (*Lawsonia inermis*). Combinations include mahalakshmi vilas rasa, vasant malti, sarvajwar harloh goldwala, satopladi churna, gilosattva, and godhanti. Other remedies consist of: clove oil with honey and garlic at bed time; ginger with honey 3-4 times per day; tulsi extract with ginger and honey; 3-4 peppers chewed slowly in mouth; cardamom powder 3 times per day; turmeric and uncooked honey three times a day; ginger and turmeric tea every four hours; and one quarter teaspoon pippali with honey three times a day. Treatment focuses on dosha-specific diet and herbs. For cough and sore throat drink tea made out of ginger, clove and cinnamon, suck a whole clove, gargle with water containing turmeric powder and salt. **Cold and flu** are kapha diseases that can be treated with lemon, gotu kala, basil, cloves and fresh ginger, taken with honey, inhaling eucalyptus fumes, and applying eucalyptus oil or ginger paste to the sides of the nose, steam bath and sauna. To treat **Sinus congestion,** mix two drops of ginger juice with one drop of fresh lime juice, half a pinch of sugarcane juice, and warm water. Put one drop in each nostril twice a day, massage the face and sinus area vigorously with a little warm sesame oil and apply a hot towel or water bottle to the sinus area. Sniff slowly and deeply, again place a hot towel over sinus area, and apply ghee inside the nostrils. Daily sinus cleaning is recommended with the aid of a concoction made out of sixteen ounces of water, one half inch of grated ginger, one tea spoon full of licorice powder, one quarter tea spoonful of pippali, and one quarter teaspoon of vacha. Boil these to one fourth of the original, add four ounces of sesame oil, and boil till all water is gone. Apply two drops in each nostril and inhale deeply. It is important to warm the oil before application. Allopathy indiscriminately uses a combination of antibiotics, anti-inflammatory drugs, steroids, chemical decongestants, and vasoactive products.

General Immunity: The concept of immunity, *Vyadhiksamatva* or *Bala*, literally means 'resistance' (*ksamatva*) against disease (*vyaadhi*) in general (*Sushruta samhita, Sutrasthana, 15:24*). **Bala**, the vitality principle, imparts firmness to the muscles, improves voice and complexion and fortifies motor and sensory functions. Bala is classified into 3 types: *Sahaja*: congenital or natural; *Kalaja*: depends upon time, season, and age; *Yuktikruta*: acquired. Factors that influence bala are: uterine health of the mother, nutrition after birth, constitution (kapha constitution has stronger immunity than pitta and vata constitutions), and mind (positive thinking increases ojas). Right karma and meditation strengthen overall immunity as do many herbs: ashwagandha, shatavari, brahmi, amalaki, garlic, guduchi, tulsi, licorice root, shankhapushpi, vacha, mandukaparni, jyotismati, jatamansi, kapikachchhu, and yastimadhu. Compounded formulae include chyawanprash, arogyavardhini, balasava rihat rasa, chintamani, and triphala. The immunity can be enhanced by various combinations of milk, ghee, honey, spices (cumin, ginger, fennel, coriander, turmeric, pepper), and pomegranate or poppy seed Chutney. Regular exercises like yoga, jogging, walking, swimming, and daily oil massage promote immunity. In modern Allopathy, decreased immunity has been related to the lack of Vitamin D, dihydroepiandrostenedione and steroid hormones, so the treatment is a combination of these constituents.

Infections, Fever and Injuries. High fever with burning sensation, thirst, red tongue, yellow coating, red eyes, perspiration, yellow urine and stool are all pitta disorders whereas vata fevers are irregular with severe pain, while kapha fevers are low grade with loss of appetite and taste along with excess salivation. Bitter herb combinations such as trikatu, dry ginger, lemon with honey, butter or ghee are used for Kapha, Pitta and Vata, respectively. Gypsum and Godanti bhasma are used to bring down very high fevers along with warm water, teas and kichri. Chronic low grade fevers can be treated with aloe gel, shatavari, guduchi, amalaki, and chyavana prash. Natural antibiotics include katuka, chiretta, gentian and barberry. Turmeric is excellent for traumatic injuries and aloe gel is also highly recommended; healing is stimulated by ginger, cayenne, sassafras, and saffron. Allopathic treatment consists of antibiotics, analgesics, and antipyretics like aspirin.

Nervous System Diseases. These are described as *Vatavyadhi* or *vata* diseases but other doshas could also be vitiated. Under this category are grouped insanity, alcoholism, addiction, and toxicomania. Treatment consists of eliminating the etiological factor (s), panchakarma, herbal nervine tonics and sedatives, meditation, pranayama and yoga. **Headaches** can be treated with ginger paste applied to the forehead, and drinking cumin-coriander tea. **Insomnia:** perform warm sesame oil massage on soles of the feet, forehead, or the whole body. Retire early, drink wine, eat heavy foods containing meat, milk and honey, listen to relaxing music, and apply sandalwood paste over the eyes. Yoga asanas are recommended but not aerobics. Also, perform meditation on the heart or breath, and chant mantras like Ram or Sham. Allopathy advises detoxification, anxiolytics, sedatives and psychotherapy.

Obsesity: Charaka described it as '*Medoroga*' and defined it as "*an invidual whose increased adipose and muscle tissues make his hips, abdomen and breasts pendulous, and whose vitality is much less than his body size, should be cared as one whose fat tissue is diseased (Medrogi) or is obese (Sthula)*". Here, ama lowers the Agni in the adipose tissues thereby blocking the channels while aggravating vata and kapha, leading to the diseases commonly associated with obesity. Vata is pacified by sudation, sauna, anuvasan basti followed by niruha basti, and herbs (triphala, guggul and shilajit). To alleviate kapha, perform an external massage with agaru, ginger, calamus, and mustard. Ama is eliminated by trikatu, guduchi, turmeric, cyperus, triphala, barberry and gentian. Fat metabolism is stimulated by pungent, bitter and astringent herbs, exercise, massage and yoga according to the VPK prakriti. Allopathic treatment is primarily based upon the intake of low calorie diet, or intake of artificial food that cannot be digested, along with exercise.

Reproductive tract Diseases. Male sexual debility is a vata disorder to be treated by tonification with ghee, nuts, lotus seeds, garlic, onion, okra, artichokes, shellfish and meat. Tonic herbs for **male sexual debility** include ashwagandha, shatavari, bala, cuscuta, and licorice, all of which are also good for male sterility. Enlarged prostate is a vata disorder and can benefit from ashwagandha, shilajit, guggul and gokshura. Herpes is largely a pitta disorder that can be helped by gotu kala and dosha specific therapies. **Menstrual disorders** are treated with regimens to balance the humors but shatavari is the main female reproductive tonic; a mixture of turmeric, cinnamon, ginger, cayenne, pippali, basil, dill, fennel, cardamom and asafoetida can be taken with aloe vera gel. **Amenorrhea** (delay or absence of bleeding) is treated with myrrh while cyperus is excellent for **dysmenorrhea** (painful bleeding). **Menorrhagia** (excessive bleeding) is treated with anti-pitta diet and astringent herbs. **Leucorrhea** is primarily a kapha disorder where local washings are done with alum, turmeric, aloe gel and licorice, along with a dosha-specific therapy. **Menopause** can be managed by pitta and vata pacifying diet (avoid salt, sugar and fermented foods) and lifestyle, along with one tea spoon full each of ashwagandha, shatavari and amalaki, aloe gel twice a day, for at least three months. Drink tea made from fresh ginger root, fennel seeds, licorice powder and cumin powder combined with abhyanga massage and pranayama. **Female infertility** is treated with tonics: shatavari, ashwagandha, aloe gel, saffron, licorice, and Dashamula. In allopathy, sexual disorders are related to the hormones produced by the endocrine glands and the treatment is to balance them.

Respiratory Tract Dysfunctions. The lungs and stomach are primary seats of kapha; phlegm is produced in the stomach, accumulates in the lungs, and then travels throughout the body. Emesis is the main therapy for kapha disorders however vata and pitta can also influence the respiratory system. Pranayama should be considered a long term therapy for lung disorders with regular breathing (exhalation twice the length of inhalation), *soham* breathing (*so* inhalation and *ham* exhalation) and alternate nostril breathing. **Asthma** is a severe form of cough that involves gasping, wheezing and difficult breathing, due to allergies and hereditary factors; bronchodilating herbs are smoked during attacks and pulmonary tonics (ashwagandha, shatavari, chyavan prash) are given to strengthen the lungs. Licorice and ginger tea is good for asthma while turmeric is good for allergic asthma. **Pneumonia** is a severe form of bronchitis treated with shringa bhasma and godanti bhasma. Antibiotic herbs include Echinacea, goldenseal, katuka and isatis, to be combined with tonifying herbs like ashwagandha, shatavari, and chyavana prash. **Allergic rhinitis** is generally a vata disorder but pitta and kapha types exist. It is treated like the common cold along with tonification using ashwagandha, bala, brahma rasayana and chyavana prash. Essential oils like menthol, eucaluptus, camphor, and ginger paste can also be applied to the temple and the nose while triphala ghee or just ghee can be applied to the eyelids. In Allopathy, antibiotics are combined with steroids and vasoactive products for the symptomatic relief of these symptoms.

Skin Afflictions: The skin has a surface area of approximately 2 sq kilometers and is the largest organ. Poor diet, poor state of circulatory and excretory systems, and elevated sugar, all lead to the build up of toxins that are the root cause of skin eruptions. Urticaria in Ayurveda is known as *sheetpitta* due to disturbed vata and kapha; in combination with disturbed pitta they create redness, swelling and itching. A predominance of bad bacteria in the gut over good bacteria leads to skin conditions like **psoriasis, rosacea, acne** etc. Regular Yoga, pranayama, and internal cleansing, will cure skin without the need for any external aid. Massage with coconut oil, or 'Doob' (grass) mixed with turmeric powder, helps to relieve **itching**. Arugampul (*Cynodon dactylon*), also known as Bermuda grass, paste along with a turmeric, will clear most of the skin diseases, blemishes, boils, itching etc. Aavarai (*Cassia auriculata*), or Tanner's Cassia flowers, can provide a radiant and glowing skin; a decoction of fresh flowers, or powder of the dried flowers, or the fresh flowers themselves, cure body heat, body odor, and salt deposits on body. Ginger juice mixed with water, giloy, turmeric, neem, dhanvyas syrup, rasmanikya, gandhak rasayana, manjisthadi churna, raktapittantaka rasa, sheetpittbhanjan rasa, khadirarisht, haridrakh, kaishore gugglu, arogyavardhani, khadar, haridrakhanda, moti pishti, kesar kasturi and gold mixed with ghee, are recommended as well. Psoriasis responds to panchagrhatta gokul (tablets or with ghee) whereas dry skin can be helped by sarwadhya rishta. Ghee, kept in a copper vessel with water for a month (Shatodhra ghee), is excellent for skin diseases as is saffron, moti bhasma, and turmeric cream. Premature **baldness** is to be treated with scalp massage using warm sesame oil, bhringaraj oil and brahmi oil, along with nasya and herbs such as gotu kala, ashwagandha, amalaki, bakuchi, sandalwood and licorice. **Boils** are treated with onion poultice, ginger powder and turmeric. **Burns** can be soothed with aloe vera containing turmeric; ghee or coconut oil may also be used. While the traditional medicine works on attacking the cause, **modern medicine works by attacking the effect**. Strong medicines and steroid-based ointments act as suppressants and at best provide only temporary relief. Mercantilism has all but taken over the practice of Dermatology in the West as women want to appear attractive and young. Consequently, manufacturers are churning out more and more products, some based on ancient Ayurvedic formulations.

Sexology: Ayurveda recognizes the extreme importance of sex in human life and sexology was called *Vajikarana*, derived from *vaji* (horse) and *karana* (to do). *Vajikarana* thus means to make oneself strong like a horse in sex Life. Herbal aphrodisiacs include: garlic, onion, almonds, dates, figs, carrots, apples, honey, milk, kamchunamati rasa, shukramatraka bati, viryasthamban bati, akarkara, kancha beej, abhrak, shilajit, ashwagandha, svedha musli, tulsi, shatavari, and jatmanasi. Massage of genital marma point on the underside of the penis, combined with simultaneous *ashwani mudra*, diamonds, padmasana, recitation of AUM, Zinc (50 mg daily), B-complex supplement, all are believed to increase sexual potency. Western medical practice uses products like

Viagra to treat erectile dysfunction that does nothing to enhance vitality though testosterone therapy is recommended in old male subjects.

Urinary Tract Diseases: Kidneys can be strengthened by spring water (chlorination is bad) or water left in a copper vessel overnight. Shilajit (500 mg to 1 g) is the best herb to vitalize the kidneys whereas dysuria can be treated with gokshura and dosha-specific therapy. Urinary tract infections stem from high pitta to be treated with sandalwood, shilajit, coriander, punarnava, lemon grass and fennel, along with dosha-specific therapy. Allopathy relies on antibiotics exclusively to kill bacteria but does not treat the underlying organ deficiency.

15.

Ayurveda Pharmacopeia

The word *bhesaja* (medicine) is derived from *bhisaj* 'healer'. Ayurveda believes that all substances found in nature have some medicinal value whose purpose is not to suppress the illness but to balance the factors in the body. Ayurvedic pharmacology is a vast science including thousands of medicines made from animals, herbs, gems, minerals, metals and colors. Dorothy Chaplin summarizes:

> **Long before the year 460 BC, in which Hippocrates, the father of European Medicine was born, the Hindus had built an extensive pharmacopeia** and had elaborate treatises on a variety of medical and surgical subjects".

Meat was freely prescribed as were other ingredients of animal origin that have to be purified by individual processes before being used for medicinal purposes. With the rise in vegetarianism, pharmacological products of animal origin have largely been abandoned. Ayurvedic pharmacology is based upon **rasya, virya** and **vipak** that are applied not only to foods but also to gems, stones, minerals, metals, color, and even to the mind and emotions. In general, sweet and salty tastes have sweet *vipak*, sour taste has sour *vipak* and pungent, bitter and astringent tastes have pungent *vipak*. All of these directly influence the doshas and dhatus. The Sanskrit texts display an impressive attempt to classify the plant world based on morphology and medicinal properties, as summarized by vanRheede in *Hortus Malabaricus*. Writers and compilers of Ayurvedic literature such as Charaka, Sushruta, Vagabhatta, Bhav Mishra, Shaligram and others have written about the qualities, characteristics and medicinal uses of the herbs, mineral, metals, chemicals, animal parts, cooked food articles, natural foods, fruits etc. Among them, the *Bhav Prakash Nighantu*, written by Bhav Mishra and *Nighantu part* (Ayurvedic Materia Medica) of the Bhav Prakash, are particularly detailed. The medicinal herbs are classified according to the nature, effects, and curative properties, as observed by the Ayurvedic practitioners. Herbal medicines need to be taken at specific times, in correct doses, and by appropriate routes.

Water is personified as the immortal medicine, brought by a chariot, known by Matali and put into them by Indra (AVS1.4.4 and 11.6.23; RV 1.23.19). Soma is also said to have declared that water is medicine for every disease (RV 1.23.2). The ritual *sutras* describe a recipe for the purification by water that dates back to the times immemorial (RV 10.137.6; AVS 6.91.3 etc). Water was considered the single most important element for the cure of internal diseases *ksetriya*, *rapas* and *amiva*. AVS 6.24 focuses on the healing properties of water as follows:

> *Indeed may the divine waters, (which) flow from the Himavant (and form) a confluence somewhere in the Sindhu, bestow on me that medicine against hrddyota (chest pain).*

> *May the waters, best healers among healers, eradicate all that which has afflicted (me) in my two eyes, in (my) two heels and in the front of (my) two feet.*

> *You, who are all the rivers which have Sindhu as husband and king, bestow on us the medicine for that (disease, and) by means of it, may we gain your benefit.*

> *The waters (are) indeed medicinal; the waters (are) the amiva-dispellers (and) the waters (are) medicines for every (disease). (Therefore) let them (be) medicine for you.*

Organics

People had a high esteem for their flora and in some rituals practice hymn to Rudra had to be muttered for six months in constant praise for herbs AVS 8.7 and RV 10.97, as translated by Frawley:

> *Plants, which as receptacles of light were born three ages before the Gods, I honor your myriad colors and your seven hundred natures.*

> *A hundred, oh Mothers, are your natures and a thousand are your growths. May you of a hundred powers make whole what has been hurt.*

> *Plants, as Mothers, as Goddesses, I address you. May I gain the energy, the light, the sustenance, your soul, you are the human being.*

> *Where the herbs are gathered together like kings in an assembly, there the doctor is called a sage, who destroys evil, and averts disease.*

> *As they fell from Heaven, the plants said, "the living soul we pervade, that man will suffer no harm".*

> *The herbs which are in the kingdom of the Moon, many fold with a hundred eyes, I take you as the best of them, for the fulfillment of wishes as peace to the heart.*

> *The plants which are queens of Soma, spread over all the Earth, generated by the Lord of Prayer, may your energy combine within this herb.*

Charaka has detailed **fifty therapeutic actions of herbs**; each group containing ten herbs is called a *Mahaashya*. In plants, vata is concentrated in the flowers and leaves, kapha in the roots, and pitta in the essential oils, resins and sap. As different plants have different concentrations of VPK, they can be used to alter body's proportion of VPK. Plants underwent three successive stages before being used as a medicine. First, they had to be acquired from their natural habitat based upon a certain morphology, fully appreciated in various hymns (AVS 8.7.4, 9, 13, 20, 23, 27; RV 10.97.2, 3, 5, 7, 9, 15, 18, 19, 21), on days ruled by Moon or Jupiter (Mondays and Thursdays), by one in a good state of mind, who is clean, facing the sun, silent, and has paid homage in his heart to Shiva. Autumn was the best time as the plants were full of sap: such that root, bark, milky sap, flower or fruit could all be used. Plants thus collected were pulverized, decocted, or concocted into medicines (AVS 8.7.5, 18, 22; RV 10.97.21), fashioned into amulets (AVS 8.7.14), and as companions of the charm (AVS 8.7.7; RV 10.97.14). The herb was personified, divinized and looked upon as a general luck-bringer (RV 10.97.4, 5, 6, 8.17; AVS 8.7.2, 19, 20). *Arundhati* was by far the most beneficial herb described as perennial, harmless, life-giving, with a honey-sweet flower (AVS 8.7.6). In other hymns, she is described as healer of severed bone, triumphant, steadfast, delivering and mender. The herbs were purified by *Khalavi, Parpati, Kupi* or *Kupipakva bhavanas* (procedures). Indus seals depict trees as plant divinities and some hymns describe the fire altar to be constructed specifically for healing purposes. *Sarngdhara* says that preparations are to be made at dawn, using root, in equal quantity, in clay pots, with water or sesame oil. Herbal preparations begin to lose potency after a year, a powder after two months, pills after one year, and ghee and oils after four months. Herbs can be potentiated with mantras, gems, gem tinctures but it is difficult to relate ancient measures and weights to the modern ones.

Amaroli (urine therapy)

Urine therapy was first described in the *Damar Tantra* and passed down orally after recitation by Shiva to Parvati. Here, a section of 107 verses details the technique and benefits of amaroli which is also mentioned in Ayurvedic treatises like *Yogaratnaakaram, Sushruta Samhita, Bhava Prakasha Ashtanga Sangraha,* and *Dhaamara Tantra* under the heading of *Shivaambu kalpa vidhi.* Recent books on the subject include *The Golden Fountain* by Coen van der Kroon and *Amaroli* by Sw. Shankadevanda of the Satyananda Yoga Academy. Dr John Armstrong revolutionized the concept of natural urine therapy and re-established its scientific validity in his book, *The Water of Life.* References to the use of urine for medicinal purposes can also be traced to ancient Egyptian, Chinese, Aztec, and Proverbs 5:15 in the Bible: *"Drink water from thy own cis-*

tern and the streams of thy own well". In recent years, interest in amaroli has received, as evident by international conferences on the subject.

All of us commence life in the womb where we float in the **Amniotic Fluid** whose main component is the **fetal urine in the womb.** Urine is a sterile fluid containing thousands of vital biochemicals, manufactured mostly at night, and any excess over the requirement of the body is removed by the kidneys. Urine contains the excess ojas that the body cannot store along with enzymes, salts, essential nutrients, hormones, urea, electrolytes etc. By drinking the **midstream morning urine**, the vital biochemicals and **ojas** are placed in the digestive system for use during the day. Urine is not a waste product which is eliminated through the skin, lungs and digestive system. It has been experimentally shown that urine destroys viruses (rabies and polioviruses) as well as bacteria that cause tuberculosis, typhoid, gonorrhea, dysentery. Clinical trials have shown that urine is useful in treating cold, flu, cancer, gout, osteoporosis, impotence, obesity, asthma, bums, tuberculosis, blisters, cuts, wounds, cataract, coughs and colds, constipation, diabetes, eczema, gangrene, heart disease, hyperacidity, diseases of the stomach and intestines, pulmonary tuberculosis, psoriasis, piles and ringworm, uterus inflammation and stiffness of the vertebral column. Dr. Dharmadhikari of the Bihar School of Yoga has ascribed the efficacy of urine to immune enhancement, aura reinforcement, prana replenishment, and as an 'elixir' that confers longevity. Amaroli mobilizes toxins within the body and the immune system attacks them which can lead to side effects like inflammation, fever, and eruptions etc that disappear when all toxins have been removed.

Urine passed at any time of the day may be drunk but the best urine is the mid-stream jet passed just after getting up in the morning which should be drunk immediately, followed by a little water, but food should be avoided for at least one half hour thereafter. Constitution determines the effects of Amaroli, vata and pitta types get excellent results, but kapha types may not notice much change and only need to do it occasionally. Teenagers, menopause women, and those over 40 years will also benefit greatly. Ayurveda and Yoga greatly increase the effectiveness of Amaroli, by loading up the urine with ojas, removing toxins from the body, increasing and distributing prana, and controlling tejas. Yogis are encouraged to drink their own urine between 4 and 6 AM as the hormones facilitate a meditative state when the mind is less inclined to wander, spiritual energy is kept high, and passage to Samadhi is smoother. Amaroli could well have been the basis of Soma practice where right foods and herbs in the diet can modify the urine to achieve altered states.

Externally, urine is used to bathe the skin and treat infections, wounds, and skin diseases. Urea present in urine seems to be a tonic for the skin and is used in many cosmetics. *Damar Tantra* recommends urine that has either been boiled to 25% of its original volume, or aged for 4-8 days in a dark bottle; massage with fresh urine can cause burns. The whole body can be massaged or just the acupressure points. The urine is left on the skin for as long as possible, even overnight, and then washed off with warm water. Soaps, shampoos etc. are to be avoided when doing urine massage but sesame oil may be applied to dry skins for extra protection. The body will smell pleasant, feel clean and rejuvenated.

The original scriptures of Ayurveda consider **cow urine to be the elixir of life**. Cow urine contains nitrogen, sulphur, phosphate, sodium, manganese, carbolic acid, iron, silicon, chlorine, magnesium, melic, citric, citric, succenic, calcium salts, Vitamins A, B, C, D, E, minerals, lactose, enzymes, creatinine, hormones and acids, all of which are needed in small amounts by the human body to balance the doshas. Whenever people urinate, these micronutrients are flushed out of the body and cow urine restores them. Cow urine is an excellent germicide and improves immunity. Some of the diseases proven to be cured by cow urine include: cough, dysmenorrhea, migraine, headache, constipation , thyroid dysfunction, skin diseases like eczema, ringworm, and itching, acne, and even AIDS. Cow urine is also believed to lower cholesterol, relieve tension, improve memory, enhance liver function, slow aging, strengthen brain and heart, destroy the toxic effects of drug residues in the body, enhance immunity, eliminate toxic substances, and maintain the digestive fire.

Herbals

Ajwain (*Apium graveolans*). Many medical properties are assigned to ajwain: it prevents bad breath, reduces toothache, calms sore throat, provides relief from bronchitis and asthma, fights indigestion, prevents flatulence; is anti-emetic and laxative; is beneficial in heart diseases, paralysis, abdominal pain, liver diseases, weakness in limbs, renal malfunction, mouth pile, in removing stones in urine and in controlling hiccups.

Alfalfa (*Medicago sativa*): stringent, slightly bitter, anti-vata and anti-kapha, anti-inflammatory, analgesic; used to treat arthritis, rheumatism, colitis, ulcers and anemia.

Aloe vera (*Aloe spp*). *Ghrit Kumari* in Sanskrit, aloe is a member of the lily family and is very cactus-like. There are over 240 species of aloe, however only 3 or 4 of them have medicinal properties; the most potent one is *Aloe vera barbadenis*. These fatty leaves contain the clear healing gel which is 96% water. The other four percent consists of 75 known substances including Vitamins A, B, C, E, calcium, amino acids, and enzymes. The gel is anti-vata, anti-pitta and anti-kapha, a powerful blood purifier, benefits liver, gallbladder, stomach, ulcers, colitis, vaginitis and cervicitis, burns, cuts and traumatic wounds. To treat vaginal herpes, mix two tea spoons of aloe vera gel with two pinches of turmeric and apply locally.

Amla. (*Emblica officinalis*) is commonly called *amlaki* in Bharata and Indian gooseberry in English. It is indicated in almost every disease and lauded in *Charak Samhita* as a magic herb. World-renowned *Chyavanprash* contains more than 50% fresh amla as it rejuvenates the whole body, delays cell aging, smooths away the wrinkles and makes the skin glow. Amla is endowed with *sheet* (cold) *virya* potency and is *guru* (heavy) as well as *ruksh* (dry). Amla contains five *rasas*: *madhur, amal, katu, tickt and kashaya*, along with ascorbic acid, phyllembin, phyllemblic acid, gallic acid, ellagic acid, zeatin, Z riboside, Z nucleotide, and tannins which retard the oxidation of Vitamin C. Pectin decreases cholesterol, inhibits platelet agglutination; its hematinic and lipolytic functions help counter diseases like scurvy and jaundice. It regulates digestion, controls acid secretion in the stomach, is beneficial in liver related disorders, retards premature graying, enhances hair and nail growth, improves eyesight, cleanses mouth, nourishes the teeth and bones, promotes peristaltic movement of the gastro intestinal tract. Amla helps in normalizing blood sugar due to the presence *of katu, tickt* and *kashaya rasa* and also helps the synthesis of insulin. It has a well proven anti bacterial, anti viral, anti fungal, nematacidal and anti protozoal actions. It exerts hypotensive action and is highly indicated in ulcers, inflammations, constipation, diarrhea, and heart burns or hyperacidity. An excellent pitta dosha suppressant, it also relieves burning sensations in palm and soles, and exerts antipyretic action. Due to the presence of *kashaya rasa, Amla* is said to enhance red blood cell production, reduce eye inflammations, and improve near sightedness.

Arjuna. (*Terminalia arjuna)* is a deciduous tree above 60 feet high, found abundantly on the Indian subcontinent. The bark can be used in the powder form or as an extract, and contains tannins, terpenoid saponins such as arjunic acid, arjunolic acid, arjungenin, flavinoids, phytosterols, calcium, magnesium, copper and zinc. The extract exerts a hypolipidemic and cholesterol reducing properties, strengthens the heart, and is used to treat ischemic heart disease, angina, myocardial infarction, cardiac arrhythmia, and congestive heart failure.

Asafetida (*Ferula asafoetida*) is a gum commonly called *Hing* which is widely used as a spice and to make pickles. It is an expectorant, laxative, kindles Agni, removes toxins, relieves stomach pain, indigestion, gastritis, flatulence, releases the locked-up gas from the abdomen, and alleviates respiratory infections, cough, chest congestion, phlegm, whooping cough, bronchitis, impotence, asthma and wheezing. It is used commonly with other herbal mixtures such as honey, dry ginger, onion juice, juice of tulsi, and betelnut juice.

Ashok (*Saraca indica*) or flame of the forest is believed to be the tree under which Buddha was born. The bark contains the estrogenic compound ketosterol which has a stimulating effect on the endometrium. Bark extract enhances general immunity and resistance in the body.

Ashwagandha. (*Withania somnifera*) has a long medicinal history going back 4000 years. *Ashwagandha* in Sanskrit means "horse's smell", probably due to the odor in its root which resembles that of a sweaty horse. In Tamil, it is called *Amukkrang Kilangu* (*Amukkara* = suppressing; *Kilangu* = root product). The alkaloids and withanoloids in the plant fight inflammation, stimulate the immune system, increase memory, alleviate infections, tremors, arthritis, increase the production of bone marrow and semen, reverse the aging process, regulate the HPA axis and the neuroendocrine system In Ayurveda, the fresh roots are sometimes boiled in milk, prior to drying, in order to leach out undesirable constituents. The berries are used as a substitute for rennet to coagulate milk in cheese making. Many international pharmaceutical companies have recently taken patents based upon the Ayurvedic knowledge of this plant.

Baking soda. Facilitates cooking, relieves acidity, gas and indigestion, helps circulation and makes skin soft, relieves rash, hives and skin infections.

Bala (*Sida cordifolia*) is used to treat bronchial asthma, cold, flu, chills, headache, nasal congestion, and fat loss.

Bhringaraj (*Eclipta alba*) is used as a restorative and rejuvenative medicine for the treatment of night blindness, syphilis, prevention of repeated miscarriage, abortion and to relieve post delivery uterine pain. Mixed with amla, coconut oil, and sesame oil, it is used for hair conditioning and hair rinse.

Bibhitaki (*Terminalia belerica*) is a tonifying and warming herb used for the treatment of dysentery and intestinal parasites, to cleanse and nourish the bodily tissues, and to balance all three doshas.

Brahmi or Gotu kola (*Bacopa monnieri*). Brahmi has been a standard medicine in Ayurveda to relieve stress, sinus problems, congestion, calm the mind, develop memory, intelligence, higher consciousness, learning, mental energy, and is also used to treat epilepsy.

Calamus (*Acorus calamus*). Root extract is an expectorant, emetic, anticonvulsive, antidote for marijuana, improves memory, emetic, relieves vata and kapha disorders.

Cardamom (*Eletarria cardamomum*). Aromatic, astringent, refreshing, enkindles digestive agni, relieves gas and pain, sharpens the mind, opens nasal passages, strengthens the heart and lungs.

Castor oil (*Ricinus communis*). Laxative, antirheumatic, relieves pain in sciatica, back and muscle. Tea is a decongestant, anti-arthritic, anti-inflammatory, and used for gout.

Cayenne pepper (*Capsicum fruitscens*). Enkindles agni, enhances circulation, causes sweating, destroys worms and parasites. Good for vata and kapha disorders and to reduce heaviness in cooked food.

Cinnamon (*Cinnamomum zeylonica*). Aromatic, stimulant, antiseptic, astringent, detoxifying, a natural cleanser, relieves vata and kapha disorders, enkindles agni, promotes digestion, relieves common cough and cold along with ginger, clove and cardamom.

Clove (*Syzgium aromaticum*). Aromatic, hot, pungent, oily and sharp; aggravates pitta but controls vata and kpaha. A natural pain reliever, it alleviates cough, congestion, colds and sinus problems.

Coriander (*Coriandrum sativum*). Greens are called cilantro and seeds coriander. Aromatic, cool, with anti-pitta properties, it is used for hoves and dermatitis, and as an aid in digestion. Coriander tea is prepared by boiling seeds in water for a few minutes and the decoction helps to cure mouth ulcers and swellings, blood cholesterol levels, diarrhea, as eyewash, and to reduce irritation and burning sensations. The juice of coriander is also used for treating nausea, morning sickness, colitis, liver disorders, peptic disease and dysentery, body fever, respiratory tract infections and cough.

Cumin (*Cumin cyminum*). Bitter and pungent, helps digestion, controls diarrhea and dysentery, relieves pain and abdominal cramps, very effective for pitta and kapha disorders.

Flax (*Linum usitatissimum*) **seeds.** laxative, decongestant, relieve constipation, distension and discomfort.

Garlic (*Allium sativum*). Sushruta recommends garlic as a universal remedy for a multitude of common ailments. The mythical origin of garlic was mentioned in forty three verses in the Bower manuscript and also in mini-treatises by Kashyapa and Vegabhata. When the king of demons drank the elixir of immortality obtained from the churning of the sea, Vishnu cut off his head but some drops from the wind pipe of the severed head fell on earth and gave birth to the garlic plant. Mentioned exclusively in Ayurveda texts, it is aromatic, hot, bitter and pungent, relieves gas, congestion, dry cough, sinus headaches, tooth aches, ear pain garlic oil, aphrodisiac, rekindles Agni, regulates the whole digestive tract and colic, ensures smooth circulation, flatulance, fertility problems, eliminates intestinal worms and parasites. Garlic is anti- vata, anti-pitta and anti-kapha and is used to make garlands, crushed for juice, fried, mixed with meat or barley, stewed, made into a paste, and even purified through a cow that had been kept three nights without grass and then fed garlic; the milk, curd and ghee are then used. Mixed with ashwagandha or myrobalans, ghee and oil, garlic was used to cure whooping cough and wheezing. The active principle appears to be Allicin which lowers cholesterol levels, reduces the risk of high blood pressure, clots, and produces healthy red blood cells

Ghee. Enkindles Agni, enhances memory, intelligence, and ojas, relieves constipation, chronic fever, anemia and blood disorders, does not increase cholesterol and carries the medicinal properties of herbs with which it is mixed such as ashwagandha, brahmi, triphala for general rejuveneation and tonicity. Milk and Ghee are used as medicine to cure acidity, anemia, asthma, bilious eruption, boils on the tongue and palate, blood impurity, bleeding dysentery, burning sensation in the eyes, constipation, chronic cough, chronic fever, chilblains, dark complexion, dark freckles, diarrhea, diabetes, epilepsy, gonorrhea, gout, general debility, jaundice, nose bleeding, piles, rashes due to biliousness, insomnia, and as an excellent antidote for poisons and drugs.

Ginger (*Glycyrrhiza glabra*). Stimulant, carminative, good for *vata*, pitta and kapha, enkindles agni, stimulates digestion, assimilation and absorption of food, alleviates throat inflammation, common cold, congestion and sinus problems, body aches, and chillblains. With honey it alleviates kapha problems such as runny nose and throat congestion. Ginger water is prepared by letting hot water run over it and a bath therein is relaxing and analgesic. It gives off a warming effect that stimulates the immune system while its essential oil can be massaged into a troubled region of the body. By rubbing it into the spinal column near the kidneys the digestive system gets the full benefits of ginger.

Guduchi (*Tinospora cordifolia*). It is used to treat blood pressure, arthritis, diabetes, weight loss, stress, sexual health, asthma and allergies, stimulate digestion, and control pitta disorders like heat and inflammation

Guggul (*Mukul myrrh*). Guggul is the resin from the tree stem whose active components are Z-guggulsterone and E-guggulsterone. It lowers cholesterol, burns body fat, reduces the total lipid content of the blood, and helps to maintain a healthy HDL to LDL ratio. It is anti-inflammatory, analgesic, an immune enhancer, used for joint pain, arthritis and sciatica. It is useful in protecting the body against common cold, skin infections, dental and eye infections. Guggul has also been effectively used for the treatment of heart attacks and thyroid dysfunction. Its antioxidant activity stems from Superoxide dismutase which eliminates free radicals from the body and prevents damage to the heart muscle.

Haritaki (*Terminalia chebula*). Fruits contain a substance which has antibacterial and anti fungal properties and is an excellent vata fighter. It is beneficial in leucorrhea, chronic ulcers, pyorrhea, fungal infections of the skin, and facilitates bowel movement. Haritaki is used in combination with other herbs in Triphala which is widely employed as an anti-aging tonic, for increasing immunity, as an expectorant, and as a strong anti-mutagen. Haritaki is used in the treatment of mouth ulcers, stomatitis, asthma, cough, candidiasis, gastroenteritis, skin diseases, leprosy, rheumatic pain and fever, wounds and arthritis.

Holy Basil (*Ocimum sanctum*). The crushed thick liquid can be applied to the eyes for treatment of night blindness and inflammation. A powdered version of Holy Basil can be used to treat sensitive teeth and gums, much like toothpaste, while leaves can be chewed to promote the healing of mouth lesions and ulcers. Insect bites can be treated using the liquid from crushed holy basil while basil tea and bath soaks relieve tension and daily stress. Holy basil lowers cholesterol and, when combined with honey, salt, cloves, and lemon, is great for relieving cold, flu, upper respiratory infections, bronchitis, asthma, and cough. Holy basil can stop the nasty symptoms of food poisoning, stomach flu, as well as childhood ailments including diarrhea and vomiting, and for easy expulsion of kidney stones via the urinary tract.

Honey. Ayurveda speaks very highly of honey for a number of reasons. It reduces vata and kapha, heals internal and external ulcers, and carries the medicinal properties of herbs with which it is mixed. Excellent blood purifier, it reduces fat, alleviates cold, cough, and congestion. Honey should never be cooked.

Jatamanasi. (*Nardostachys jatamanasi*) calms the mind, pacifies palpitation, tension, headaches, restlessness and is used for treating insomnia, mental instability, and as a memory enhancer.

Karela. Bitter gourd has many medicinal properties: appetizer, antipyretic, antibilious, laxative, anti-diabetic, hypoglycemic, and insulin-like. It is used for the treatment of asthma, bronchitis, pharyngitis, rhinitis, scabies, psoriasis, ringworm infection, and mycose; it alleviates itching sensations, calms respiratory diseases, is a blood purifier, and helps to prevent liver damage due to alcoholism.

Isabgol. The husk obtained from the *Psyllium* plant cleans the gastro intestinal tract by removing the toxins associated with chronic constipation, piles, fissures and fistulas. Isabgol helps to moisten the hard stools and brings down the burning sensation after defecation, reduces strain during defecation in persons suffering from cardio vascular diseases, hernia and pregnancy.

Licorice (*Glycyrrhiza spp*). Sweet and slightly astringent, it is a natural expectorant, germicidal, antidote for peptic ulcers and gastritis. Licorice ghee is used for diabetes, bronchitis, cold, asthma, and wound healing.

Long pepper (*Piper longum*) or pippali, is the primary ingredient in Ayurveda to treat kapha disorders. Together with ginger and black pepper it is found a in a great many receipes for the treatment of a whole spectrum of disorders.

Manjishta (*Rubia cordifolium*). is probably the best blood-purifying herb in Ayurveda. It cools and detoxifies, regulates blood pressure, reduces blood vessel constriction, and reverses blood clot formation

Mustard (*Brassica alba*). Very pungent, hot, sharp, penetrating and oily, enkindles agni and neutralizes toxins but aggravates pitta. It is anallagesic, reduces muscle spasms, cooked with garlic, onion and vegetables it makes food easy to digest.

Neem (*Azadiracta indica*), antispectic, insect-repelling, used to control diabetes; many many other uses led to the patenting of several products in the US (see Neem letter).

Nutmeg (*Myristica fragrans*). Aromatic and stimulant, with milk it forms a tonic for heart and brain, as well as an aphrodisiac; also used to treat diarrhea, abdominal gas, loss of appetite and insomnia. Good for balancing vata and kapha.

Onion. (*Allium cepa*). Strong irritant and pungent due to ammonia in the vapor, stimulates senses, aphrodisiac, anticonvulsive, and relieves epileptic seizures as eye drops or nasal inhalant. It reduces cholesterol, asthma, cough, spasms, nausea, vomiting, and destroys intestinal worms. Grated onion with one half tea spoon each of turmeric and curry powder will relieve joint pain when applied as a paste to the affected area.

Opium. It was used by Sangdhara for rejuvenation: 12 g each of powdered pellitory, ginger, cube pepper, saffron, long pepper, nutmeg, cloves and sandalwood with 100 gram opium mixed into a powder and taken with one gram of honey. Lovers should use it at night for pleasure and strength.

Pepper (*Piper longum*). Pungent, hot, enkindles agni, increases digestive secretions, fights constipation and dry hemorrhoids, combats worms in the large intestine, and relieves swelling. Mixed with ghee it relieves pitta disorders such as dermatitis and hoves.

Salt. Relieves gas and distension of the abdomen, helps increase nasal drainage, aggravates pitta and kapha as well as hypertension.

Safed musli (*Asparagus adscendens*) is an aphrodisiac, stimulant, tonic, and rejuvenator.

Sarpagandha (*Rawolfia serpentina*) is well known for the control of blood pressure.

Shallaki (*Boswellia Serrata*). Contains boswellic acid which is known to combat cancer, indigestion, asthma, inflammation, and arthritis pain.

Shilajit. Asphaltum is a resinous matter that oozes out of the Himalayan Mountains during summer, and consists of plant matter decomposed due to pressure caused by sliding of the crusts. In Sanskrit shilajit means ruler of mountains, suppressor of weakness, and it improves resistance to diseases. It is consumed after purification with milk that helps to neutralize any toxins present in it. It improves immunity and is endowed with antiseptic, laxative, rejuvenation, tonic, respiratory stimulant, disinfectant, aphrodisiac and diuretic activity. Its properties like *laghu* (light), *ruksh* (dry), and *ushan* (hot) enhance *virya* potency; shilajit is helpful in suppressing vata dosha which is very much responsible for early aging and loss of energy. It provides vitamins and minerals, reverses the aging process, wrinkles and loosening of the skin. Its constituents *katu, tickt, kashaya rasa*, and fulvic acid are all antioxidants and reduce the production of free radicals as well as cell peroxidation. It is also used to cure epilepsy, obesity, kidney disorders, menstrual problems, asthma, hemorrhoids, jaundice, and sexually transmitted diseases.

Soma. It is identified as a stimulant of the *Ephedra* family by Falk but this is debatable because both Sushruta and Aitareyabrahmana describe rejuvenation by the milk from Soma plant in a Soma sacrifice ceremony which lasted four months. The rejuvenated being was so radiant that the person could not look at himself in the glass and the body could last ten thousand years. In fact, twenty four types of soma plants were described depending upon location, appellation, form and power. All of them could be recognized as having fifteen leaves, milky latex, a bulb, and tendrils. The very best Soma is the *Candramas* from Himalayas, near the Indus, but some five types could be obtained from Kashmir. There are major differences in the identification of Soma between North and South India.

Turmeric. (*Curcuma longa*) Turmeric as a specific drug is described in Charaka samhita, Sushruta samhita, Ashtanga sangraha, and the lexicons of Chakradatta and Vangasena. Turmeric is known as the "golden spice", as well as the "spice of life", and has at least 6000 years of documented history as medicine and use in many socio-religious practices. Bitter, slightly pungent, hot, light, acrid, and irritant, good blood purifier, helps digestion and relieves congestion, soothes cough, tonsils, asthma, anti-arthritic, anti-bacterial, anti-inflammatory, and anti-diabetic. Turmeric salt paste may be applied locally to alleviate traumatic swelling. It is able to reduce corpulence, stimulate all functions, clear channels; a curing agent for kapha and pitta it is very good for skin afflictions, as an enhancer of complexion, diabetes, leprosy, thirst, bleeding, elephantiasis, calculus, inflammations, anemia, and abscess. In Rajanighantu by Narahari, Haridra (turmeric) is stated to be an effective remedy for rheumatoid arthritis and itching. Nighanturatnakara (an ancient lexicon of Ayurveda) points out more actions such as anthelmintic property, anti-poisonous effects, curative property in catarrhal affections, anorexia and enlargement of neck glands.

Valerian. (*Valeriana* spp) Tagara is the leading tranquilizer product in Europe, mainly used for treating nervous headaches, irritability, epilepsy, hysteria, vertigo, convulsions, delirium and various other symptoms associated with nervous system, as also for treating muscle spasms, stomach cramps, nerve tension, breathlessness, wheezing, panic attacks, palpitations, emotional stress, migraine headaches, common colds, cough, and to expel phlegm from the chest and throat. The concoction or tea prepared from this drug is used for the treatment of pinworms and tapeworms.

Metals and Minerals

Rasa is a word derived from Sanskrit which has several meanings like: *"Rasyate aaswadyate iti rasa"* meaning taste, *"Rasati shariire aasu prsarati it Rasa"* meaning juice, *"Rasati aharahargachhati iti Rasa"* meaning first material formed after digestion, *"Rasanaat Sarva dhatuunam Rasaityabhdhiiyate"* meaning material which is capable to lick and digest all metals or mercury. Transmutation of base metals into gold was made possible by correct combination of mercury, sulphur and salt, and an energy called 'azoth' (prana). In Tantra, this was used as a metaphor for the attainment of pure consciousness by the correct practice of hatha yoga. As the planet Mercury is associated with the central nervous system and sense perceptions in the body, their control would permit the attainment of any desire that the mind is set upon. The source of bindu is the *Sahasrara chakra*, personified as semen in the physical body, which is compared to mercury. Significant progress in alchemy in ancient Bharata was eulogized thus by Will Durant (*Our Oriental Heritage*):

> *"Something has been said about the chemical excellence of cast iron in ancient India, and about the high industrial development of the Gupta times, when India was looked to, even by Imperial Rome, as the most skilled of the nations in such chemical industries as dyeing, tanning, soap-making, glass and cement... By the sixth century the Hindus were far ahead of Europe in industrial chemistry; they were masters of calcinations, distillation, sublimation, steaming, fixation, the production of light without heat, the mixing of anesthetic and soporific powders, and the preparation of metallic salts, compounds and alloys. The tempering of steel was brought in ancient India to a perfection unknown in Europe till our own times; King Porus is said to have selected, as an especially valuable gift for Alexander, not gold or silver, but thirty pounds of steel. The Moslems took much of this Hindu chemical science and industry to the Near East and Europe; the secret of manufacturing "Damascus" blades, for example, was taken by the Arabs from the Persians, and by the Persians from India."*

Alchemy was led by the Hindu school under Adinatha Siddha, and by Buddhist school under Nagarjuna, but compared to magic and therefore heavily censured by Christians. All metals possess tremendous healing energy but have to be purified using oil, cow's urine, milk, ghee, buttermilk, to remove all toxicity, but this has not been confirmed by modern science. As a result of the interest and investigations of Siddhas, Ayurveda "alchemy" developed, primarily using purified heavy metals combined with other unique and often very potent medicinal substances. In many Ayurveda products, heavy metal contamination with mercury, lead etc. has been documented, that can lead to poisoning, and remains a major concern; their import into many countries is therefore prohibited.

Rasayan is a Sanskrit word meaning: Path (*ayana*) of the Juice (*rasa*), or *Elixir vitae*, used to describe chemistry and alchemy; chemistry is generally called *Rasayan Shastra* in Sanskrit. *Kamya* Rasayans boost body energy, immunity and general health. *Naimittika* Rasayans help to fight a specific disease. Puri has given detailed account of classical formulations such *as Amrit Rasayana, Brahm Rasayana, Jawahar Mohra, Kamdugdha Ras, Laxami Vilas Ras, Madanoday Modak, Makrdhawaj vati, Manmath Ras, Mukta Panchamrit Rasayana, Nari Kalyan Pak, Navjeevan Ras, Navratna Ras, Navratnakalp Amrit, Panchamrit Ras, Paradi Ras, Ramchuramni Ras, Rattivalbh Pak, Shukar Amrit Vati, Smritisagar Ras, Suvarn Malini Vasant, Suvarn Vasant Malti, Swapanmehtank, Vasant Kusmakar Ras, Visha Rasaayana, Vrihda Vangeshwar Rasa*. Rasayanas for different organs include: eye (triphala, licorice, shatavari); nose (anu tail nasya); skin (tuvarak, catechu, bakuchi); brain (gotu kola, calamus); heart (gold, arjuna, guggul); neuro-muscular system (bala, garlic, guggul, nagbala).

In Ayurveda, **all matter contains the Universal Consciousness or energy** known as prana. Metals can therefore be used to heal, strengthen, and protect. When gold, silver, iron, and other heavy metals come into contact with human tissue, their electromagnetic energy 'astral light' affects the body at a cellular level by counteracting unwanted cosmic energy. This is why some people wear a silver bracelet or copper band for healing. ***Bhasmas*** are prepared by a special kind of oxidation where the metal is heated on charcoal and then dipped into oil, buttermilk, cow's urine, kanji (fermented wheat gruel) and a decoction of horse gram. The metal is heated and dipped into these mediums seven times and then sealed airtight in an earthen shell which is heated for 6-8 hours on coal from special trees or cow dung. For certain metals the whole procedure is repeated many times and the bhasmas are then tested to ascertain that they are no longer toxic. Certain bhasmas can be prepared by heating for just 6 hours. Prominent bhasmas include gypsum ash, *shankha bhasma* (conch shell), *shringa bhasma* (deer horn), silver *bhasma* and gold *bhasma*.

Copper. Copper was the first metal to be mined in the copper age some 10,000 years ago. It alleviates kapha, acts as a tonic for liver, spleen, and lymphatic system and is used to treat obesity, edema, anemia and infections; water was stored in copper vessels to curb the growth of pathogens. More recently, copper had been found to stimulate collagen production, to much delight of the cosmetic industry. A simple treatment for healing is to place a copper band around the arm.

Gold. Vedas have many references to a connection between gold and **long life**. Charaka says that no poison can be sustained in the body of people who have ingested gold whose presence destroys the effects of all types of poisons especially *Garavisa*. Evidence for the idea of transmuting base metals to gold appeared in 2nd - 5th century CE in Buddhist texts. Gold is *madhura* (sweet) and *kasaya* (astringent) in *rasa*, *snigdha* (oily) and *laghu* (light) in *guna*, *sita* (cold) in *virya*, and *madhura* in *vipak*. Its actions are *visanghna, varnya, rasayana, brimhana, rucikara, dipana, medhya, smriti vardhana*, and it is the best aphrodisiac. It inhibits wasting of the body tissue, reduces body weakness, prevents early aging, improves body complexion, is antimicrobial and antipyretic. It is used as a nervine tonic, improves memory, immunity stamina, heart muscle, lungs and spleen. Gold water is prepared by boiling a gold ornament in water until the volume is reduced to one half. The electronic energy of gold now enters the water and one tea spoon full two-three times a day will energize the heart. Gold is turned into ash by fire and *swarna bhasma* or gold ash is anti-depressant, anxiolytic, anticataleptic, nervine tonic and a good cure for rheumatoid arthritis. Gold potentiates all medicines and stimulates longevity.

Iron. Iron is an overall strengthener and rejuvenator, enhances bone marrow and red blood cell production, benefits blood circulation and anemia, increases muscle tone, fortifies nerve tissue, and opposes hepatosplenomegaly.

Lead. Very effective for the treatment of syphilis, gonorrhea, leucorrhea, and vaginal discharge.

Lapis lazuli. Produces feelings of wellbeing while expelling all doshas from the body.

Makardhvaj. This is the most potent Ayurveda rasa preparation containing sulphur, mercury, cloves, camphor, nutmeg, black pepper and gold. It is used as a heart tonic, aphrodisiac and general body rejuvenator.

Mercury. Mercury, so vital to alchemy everywhere, was first mentioned in the *Arthashastra* (ca 400 BC). Known as the semen of Lord Shiva, mercury balances all three doshas, has a soothing effect, prevents disease and old age, nourishes all of the vital parts of the body, and improves vision. It is a *vrisya* (aphrodisiac), *balya* (tonic), *snigdha* (anointing), *rasayana* (rejuvenative), *vrana sodhana* and *ropana* (wound cleaner and healer), and *krimighna* (antimicrobial). Mercury is also said to bestow a firm physique, a stable mind, and to be the best destroyer of disease. It enkindles the enzyme system, transforms and regenerates, stimulates intelligence, and awakens awareness. The potency of many drugs is believed to increase a thousand fold when used with mercury and sulphur.

Rasavatam (the way of Mercury) was a form of alchemy in early Bharata, practiced mainly with herbs, drugs, and prepared medicines, and quite different from the traditions of alchemy in medieval Europe. Sulphides of mercury were traditionally used in Rasavatam and Ayurveda to cure disease and prolong life. One such preparation is named *thanga baspam* and claimed to extend human life span. Nagarjuna is considered to be the first to use mercury for alchemic purposes as he said *"siddhe rase karisyaami nirdaridryamyaham jagat"* meaning I am experimenting with the mercury to eliminate poverty from this world. *Rasa Shastra* is based on the theory of *"yatha lohe tatha dehe"* or the science of mercury. It classifies metals, minerals, diamond, gemstones and poisons into various categories and the transformation from lower metals into higher metal through the help of mercury. Whereas alchemy involves turning mercury into gold, *rasayana* is the rejuvenation of the mind and body. Mercury was also used for the incineration of metals and minerals to eliminate toxic components and generate therapeutically usable bhasmas. Once the metal is converted into the bhasma, it should not revert into the metal by any means called *Apunarbhava*, it should be so light as to float on water called *Varitara*, its particles should be small enough to enter the lines of the palm and become invisible at the surface called *Rekha purnata*.

Silver. Silver is astringent and sour, cools pitta but is also good for vata, promotes strength and stamina. Silver ash is helpful for emaciation, chronic fever, heartburn, inflamed intestine, hyperactivity of the gallbladder. Silver water, prepared like the gold water, has the same properties; milk heated in a silver pot is beneficial as well. It gives strength to the brain, heart and stomach, fights vertigo, insanity, palpitations, pre-ejaculation, and *mada* intoxication.

Tin. Purified ash is used to treat diabetes, gonorrhea, syphilis, asthma, respiratory infection, anemia, skin disease, lung disease, lymphatic obstruction, and for rejuvenation.

Prominent Herbal Mixes

Powders have the shortest shelf life (one year), tablets are good up to two years, and medicated ghee for only six months. For weight loss and general cleansing use: Ashwagandha 2 ozs, neem 1 oz, kapilacchu 1 oz, turmeric ½ oz, myrrh 1 oz, manjistah 1 oz, ginger, 1 oz, fennel ½ oz, coriander ½ oz, cardamom ¼ oz, cinnamon ¼ oz, bala ½ oz. To maintain the doshas in balance, many preparations are available.

Asafetida compound. Asafetida, trikatu, rock salt, black cumin, ajwain (carminative, antispasmodique, stimulant, ease abdominal pain, gas, colic, and indigestion).

Ashwagnadha churna. Ashwagandha, vidari kanda (tonic, aphrodisiac, analgesic).

Avipattikar churna. Trikatu, Triphala, cyperus, vidanga, cardamom, cinnamon, cloves, trivrit, raw sugar, sometimes fortified with gold bhasma (hyperacidity, heartburn, indigestion, laxative).

Brahmi bati. Gotu kola, shankhapushpi, calamus, black pepper, various minerals (nervine tonic, memory loss, epilepsy, paralysis).

Chandranadi churna. Sandalwood, fennel, long pepper, black pepper, cloves (urinary antiseptic, cough, asthma, venereal diseases).

Chaturbija. Fenugreek, watercress, kalajaji, yavani (digestive, stimulant).

Dhatupaushtic churna. Shatavari, gokshura, cannabis seed, vamsha rochana, sarsaparilla, cubeb, mucuna, black and white musali, trikatu, dioscorea, ashwagandha, nishotha, sometimes fortified with gold bhasma (aphrodisiac, tonic, rejuvenative).

Guduchi sattva. Guduchi extract (liver and urinary disorders, fever, malaria).

Kamini vidrawan ras. Akarkara, shunuthi, lavanga, curcuma, pippali, jatiphala, shveta chandana, shuddha hingula, shiddha gandhaka, khurasani ajwain (aphrodisiac, male sexual tonic, improves quality, improves the quantity of semen and ejaculation).

Lashuandi bati. Garlic, cumin, rock salt, sulphur, trikatu, asafetida, lemon juice (distension, gas, loss of appetite, laxative).

Lavanbhaskar churna. Five salts, fennel, long pepper, black cumin, cinnamon, nagakesar, rhubarb root, pomegranate seeds, cardamom (appetite stimulant, constipation).

Mahasudarshan powder. Bitters such as chiretta, guduchi, barberry, trikatu, triphala, and cannabis (antipyretic, diuretic, splenomegaly and hepatomegaly).

Panchkola. Pippali, pippali root, chavya, chitrak, dry ginger (digestive, stimulant).

Sarasvat powder. Ashwagandha, calamus, shankhapushpi, ajwain, cumin, trikatu, rock salt (nervine tonic, epilepsy, mania).

Siddhamakardhwaj. Makardhwaj, gold bhasma, pearl bhasma. (excellent tonic, rasayana, rejuvenator).

Sitopladi churna. Rock candy, bamboo manna, long pepper, cardamom, cinnamon (antitussive, expectorant, indigestion, cold, cough, fever).

Trikatu. Dry ginger, long pepper, black pepper (stimulant, digestive).

Triphala. Haritakai, Bibitaki, Amalaki, ginger, sometimes supplemented with asafetida (laxative, rejuvenative).

Trijata. Cinnamon, cardamom, cinnamon leaf (carminative, anti-emetic).

Trimada. Vidanga, cyperus, chitrak (opens channels, clears obstructions).

Trisugandhi churna. Cinnamon, cinnamon leaf, cardamom (digestive stimulant, gas, distension).

Vasanta Kusumakar. Gold bhasma, rajat bhasma, vanga bhasma, naga bhasma, lauha bhasma, abhraka bhasma, pravala bhasma, mukta bhasma, rasa sindur. (Excellent rejuvenator, and tonic).

Other herbal combinations include the five barks (Panchavalkala), five bitters (Panchatikta), five roots (Panchamula), ten roots (dashmula), and gugguls. Ayurvedic wines are fermented herbs, the best known being Draksha, made like the grape wines. Medicated oils include **Bhringaraj taila** (bhringaraj and sesame oil) used for hair loss and as nervine tonic; **Brahmi taila** (gotu kola and other herbs in coconut oil base) used as a nervine tonic and sedative; **Chandranadi taila** (sandalwood, licorice, saussurea etc and sesame oil) used as antipyretic and sedative; **Mahanarayana taila** (shatavari, castor root, brihati, bala and sesame oil) used to treat arthritis, gout, paralysis; **Narayana taila** (shatavari, ashwagandha, bilva root, brihati, neem, dashamula, milk and sesame oil) used for rheumatic pain, paralysis and fever. Incense has been traditionally used for calming the mind and counter negative emotions, just like the essential oils, and uses dosha-specific ingredients; for general purposes, sandalwood, rose, and camphor incense may be used.

16.

World Medical Traditions

Vedic literature is vast, containing some 4524 known scriptures and **over fifty thousand manuscripts,** despite repeated loss and destruction by the invading Muslims and Christians. The rishi Krishna Dwaipayana, better known as Veda Vyasa, "*Vyasa*" meaning "editor" or "compiler", reputedly compiled the *shruti* hymns into four Vedas, each book being supervised by one of his disciples. The antiquity of the *Vedas* has been hotly debated by the opposing forces of reductionists and nationalists who provide the dates of 1700 BC or less and 3200 BC or more, respectively, for Rigveda. Each Vedic branch is divided into *Samhita, Brahmana, Aranayak and Upanishad* but for each *Veda* there are four *upavedas* (*Ayurveda, Dhanurveda, Gandharvaveda and Sthapatyaveda*). *Vedas* admit 1131 branches of which *Rigveda* has 21, *Yajurveda* has 101, *Samveda* has 1000 and *Atharvaveda* has 9. Then there are 6 *Angas*, 18 *Puranas*, 18 *Smritis*, 2 Epics, as well as *Yantras, Tantras, Mantras* and *Jantris*. To understand the Vedas, *Vedangas* were composed to deal with six special branches of knowledge: phonetics (*shiksha*), ritual (*kalpa*), grammar (*vyakalpa*), etymology (*nirukta*), metrics (*chandah*) and astronomy (*jyotisha*). In Grammar, *Ashtadhyayi* of Panini may go back to 500 BC but other grammatical works certainly existed before. *Mahbhasya* of Katayana is dated 150 BC and it comments on *Ashtadhyayi*. Philosophical *sutras*, besides *Samhitas* and *Brahamanas*, consist of several *mimamsas* (investigation): *Purvamimamsa, Uttaramimamsa* or the *Vedanta, Samkhya, Yogasutra, Nyaya* (method) and *Vaisesika. Arthashastra, Nitishastra, Dandaniti, Rajaniti,* etc that deal with practical aspects of life: administration, economics, politics, arts, techniques, mining etc. The most important, *Arthashastra* of Kautilya (also known as Chanakya), contains 6000 slokas, 150 chapters and 180 subjects, and is dated 300 BC. The *Kalpasutras* contain detailed instructions for performing rituals and are divided into *Srautasutras* (great sacrifices), *Grhyasutras* (ceremonies in the domestic life), *Dharmasutras* (religious and secular laws) and *Sulvasutras* (measurements for altars etc). Mathematical historian David Pingree has estimated that there exist: *"at present in India and outside of it some million manuscripts on various aspects of jyotishastra…neither cataloged nor translated and constitute a territory that remains remarkably unexplored"*.

No other region, religion or culture can boast of as much in quantity, quality and antiquity. The Five Classics of China go back to the first half of the 1st millennium BC: While in ancient Egypt the earliest literary activity can be dated 2755-2255 BC, most output came much later. Assyrian literature under Ashurbanipal (669-626 BC) recounted mythological poems of Sumerians e.g. Poem of Creation (Enuna Eliah) and Gilgamesh circa 2000 BC; other works imitated the ancient Sumerian or Accadian Hymns to Gods, incantations, ritual writings, genealogies of kings, victories and defeats. Persia produced the Avesta and Gatha, both religious and devotional concerning Zoroastrianism, dated 1200 BC.

Homeric poems are prayers, vows and hymns to the gods and the dead, dated 800 BC. Iliad and Odyssey recount the victories of Achilles and Odysseus over twelve maritime and eleven inland cities, via colonization by the Greeks, Troy being the twelfth of the latter. Theogony by Hesiod (700 BC) is a systematic list of divinites in time periods and generations as well as union between goddesses and mortals. Elegies, Monodic lyrics, and love poetry by Sappho go back to 700 BC and predate tragedy which evolved slowly. Roman literature does not go farther back in time than 500 BC and is limited to epic poems about the deeds of brothers Vibenna and Mastarna, and of fighting between Etruscans and Celts. The antiquity of the Old Testament is debatable because the oldest written sources go back to the Massoretic rescension 6th-11th CE. Pentateuch concerns the most obscure and the earliest periods of Hebrew life and was probably conceived around time of Moses 1300-1150 BC but took formal shape only around some 800 BC.

It is therefore clear that the **ideation of Sanskrit literature has no parallels in the world** and the theory of humors, that dominated world medicine until the 17th century, could not possibly have come from a source other than from ancient Bharata. **Hijacked by Greeks, Arabs and others**, Ayurveda eventually became Hippocratic and Yunani medicines, respectively, as developed below.

Pre-Christian healing traditions of the Druids, Greeks, Celts, Germans and Slavs had something in common with Ayurveda as well. This is well summarized by P.N. Oak in World Vedic Heritage (quoted in Knapp):

> *"Thus a close study of allopathic terminology, whether of ailments, physical organs, symptoms, remedies, or instruments will found to be based on Ayurveda because during the universal unitary Vedic administration it was only Ayurveda which was the sole medical system which was used throughout the world. With the shattering of the world medical system after the*

Mahabharata war, fragments of Ayurveda surviving in different parts of the world assumed the form of tribal remedies or as rival systems such as homeopathy and allopathy. This has a parallel in theology and religion too in as much as after the breakup of the world Vedic theology, cults of different gods and goddesses, such as Mithraism, Jainism, Judaism, Buddhism and Shaivism, not hostile or dissimilar to Vedic culture, at first cropped up. However, later even hostile and militant faiths such as Christianity and Islam made their appearance".

Oak also provided **comparison between some English and Sanskrit words**: English fever,   entrails, nasal, herpes, gland, drop, hiccups, muscle, malignant, osteomalacia, dyspepsia, surgeon, fertility, anesthesia, homeopathy, allopathy are derived from Sanskrit: jwar, antral, naas, serpes, granthi, drups, hicca, mausal, malle, asthi-malashay, dush-pachanashay, salya-jan, falati-iti, anasthashayee, samaeo-pathy, alag-pathy, respectively (further details in Knapp).

Greek and Roman

Of the Minoan medicine we know almost nothing though it dominated until about 1000 BC and later formed Greek medicine, as Greek tribes overran Minoans, the last being Troy. The cult of the serpent is ascribed to the Minoans who also derived a lot from Egypt. Homer tells us little of Medicine in Odyssey and Iliad except to mention some rudimentary human anatomy during war, wounds, bleeding, and symptoms surrounding death on the battlefield. The traditional view is that Asclepius, the Greek God of healing, was originally a Thessaly chieftain whose sons, Machaon and Podalirius, became well known physicians and fought in the Trojan war; later genealogies trace his origin to Apollo though one says that he was a local demon who dwelt in earth. Although originally traced to Egypt and Babylonia, in Greece the Aesculapius serpent became a symbol of Apollo in the sanctuaries and temples dedicated to him. It was later introduced into Rome at the time of the great plague of the 3rd century BC.

The first known Greek medical school opened at Cnidus in 700 BC where Alcmaeon authored the first anatomical work while Hippocrates established his own medical school at Cos. It is clear, however, that the Greeks imported Egyptian substances into their pharmacopoeia, and this influence became more pronounced after the establishment of a school of Greek medicine in Alexandria. Medical philosophy was the preoccupation of thinkers like Pythagoras (580-498 BC), Heraclitus (ca 500 BC), and Parmenides (450 BC), though Alcmaeon of Crotona (500 BC) was a biologist and physician. Pythagoras belonged to the Orphic school and believed in transmigration of soul, a basic preamble of the Vedic thought. Almost all of the religious, mathematical and philosophical theories taught by Pythagoreans were known in India in 600 BC or before and Pythagoreans, like Jains and Buddhists, refrained from the destruction of life and eating meat. Orphism and Indian transcendental philosophy abound in parallels. Herodotus, born 484 BC, probably used the account of Scyclax to write about India but attributed all this wisdom to Egypt whose monuments fascinated the Greeks.

Empedocles (504-443 BC) maintained that **man breathes through the pores of his body** starting from birth, that heart, not the brain, was the source of consciousness. Hippon felt that **fetal bones come from the father and muscles from the mother.** In the Greek theory of vision, the **eye was supposed to send out a beam of light** (Figure 8) on the object for perception and the theory was so adopted by the Pythagorean School, Zeno (485-430 BC), Ptolemy (2nd century BC) and Euclid (3rd century BC) although denounced by Epicurus (341-280 BC). Empedocles (491-430 BC) favored a two way transmission while Plato (428-348 BC) suggested that a divine fire or luminous force from the eye encountered the light sent by the object and this union formed the vision; the quantity of the divine fire changed one color into another. Plato further elaborated that the fluid in one eye made it sensitive to the fluid from the other eye. Theophrastus (370-285 BC) tells us that Empedocles made distinction between thought and perception and his *Historia Plantarum*, written between third and the second century BC, founded the science of botany. Theophrastus also recognized the role of sex in the reproduction of some higher plants. In the first century CE, Dioscorides wrote a compendium of more than 500 plants that remained an authoritative reference until the 17th century. Most of these absurd ideas remained unchallenged until the 11th century CE and were taken as proofs of the ancient Greek wisdom.

Plato, a philosopher and not at all a scientist or medical practioner, tells us that **the womb is an animal inside a woman** which is desirous of bearing children; **floating freely** inside the body it could damage the vital organs into which it lodges (Figure 9). Hysteria was supposed to result from the movement of the womb in the body to an area such as the heart, the cure was again sex and progeny but potions, baths, fumigations etc. were also recommended by Hippocratic authors. For Plato, the **semen resided in the brain** but under false *Eros* it was drawn down the spinal channels to the penis. Plato described channels along the sides of the spinal column which cross one another and which carry soul power. This is closely related to the imagery of *kundalini* yoga and the seven *chakras* and appears to be derived from knowledge imported from Bharata.

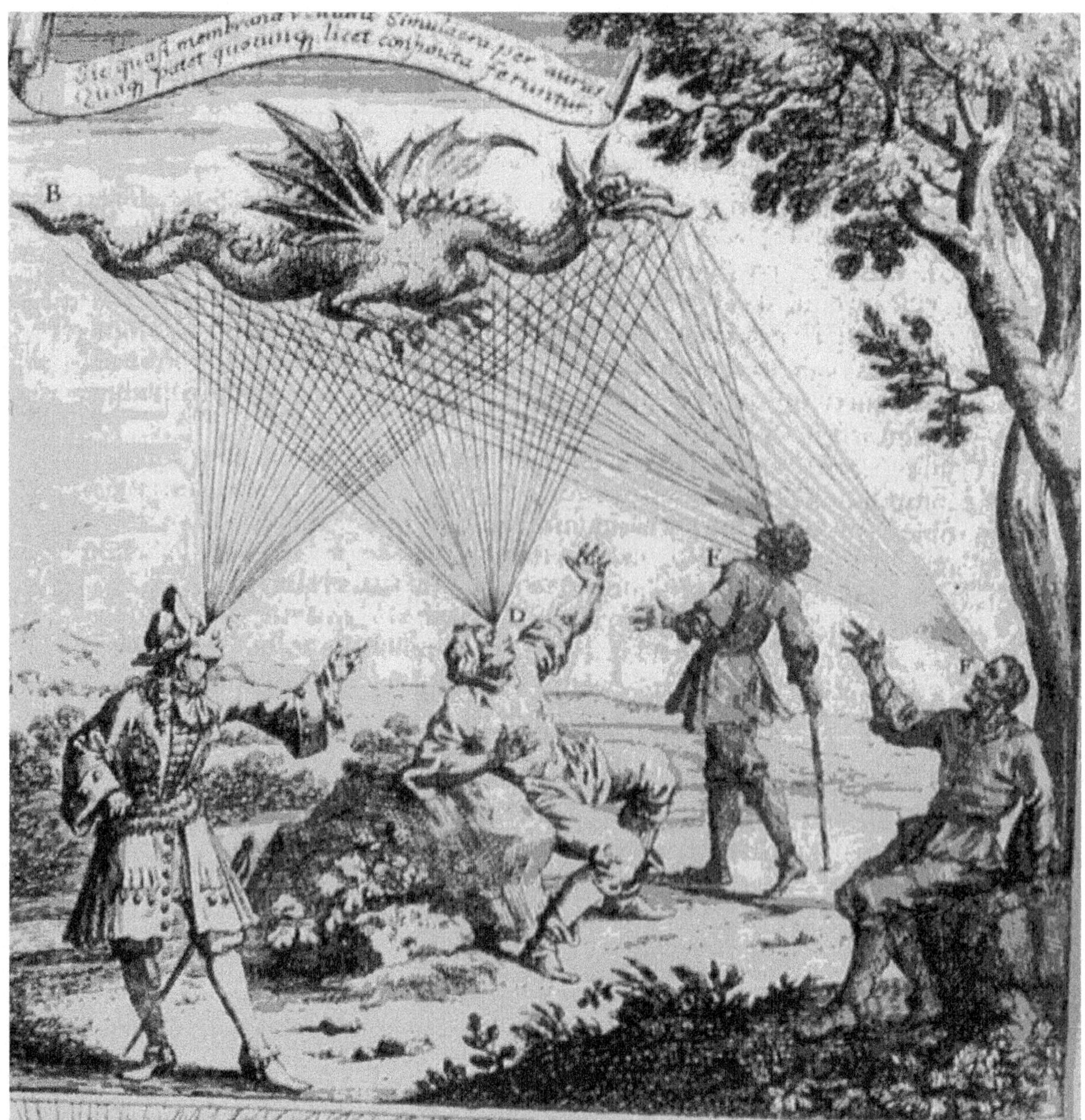

Figure 8. The Greek theory of Vision, hijacked by philosophers with no scientific or medical training, held that the eye sent a beam of light on the objects to be perceived. It is to be contrasted with cataract removal by Vedic-Buddhist surgeons 1000 BC when ocular anatomy and physiology were well advanced (taken from Alhazen by Mirshahi).

Aristotle (384-322 BC), son of a Macedonian physician, studied under Plato at Athens, but crossed over to Asia Minor after Plato's death in 347 BC to become teacher to Alexander and died a few months after the latter. Since **medical dissection was prohibited,** it was not possible to advance in anatomy/physiology. He believed that the **heart was the body's nerve center,** and could never become diseased and Galen also subscribed to this view (Figure 9). He made no distinction between arteries and veins and also disregarded the brain, in contrast to Plato. He maintained that the female contributed **only the passive material to the embryo,** chiefly from the **menstrual blood,** whereas the **father provided** the '*Homunculus*' which arose out of guiding principle from the man. In the creation of a human being, matter was supplied by the female in the form of menses; the male seed acted as the formal and efficient cause of conception, supplying the bodily shape and rational facility. Menses were an imperfect residue created when female coldness made it impossible for concoction (a sort of cooking) to take place. In males, warmth allowed concoction to occur, producing efficient seeds. The embryo that grew in the warmest part of the womb developed more fully and quickly, and thus became a male. The embryo that developed in the colder part of the womb lacked the heat to concoct fully and thus became an imperfect female. Some doctors felt that both men and women produce both types of seeds. Aristotle sums up: '*a woman is, as it were, an infertile male*' (cited in Joshel). Aristotle, in contrast to earlier philosophers, placed the rational soul in the heart, rather than the brain. The woman is less hot than man and therefore incapable of effecting the final transformation which gives rise to sperm. Thus, the role of woman was passive. Homosexuality was a waste of sperm and even dangerous, but he did not condemn it outright as immoral.

Aristotle found females incipiently monstrous, redeemed only by the natural reproductive utility of the womb. Aristotle also believed that **hair grew from the moisture provided by semen** in man's head and that women also possessed semen but far less so than men. As another proof of superiority of men to women, Aristotle claimed that **men had more teeth** (see Mayhew and Toohey, and Marks, for more details). He held that the female constitution was inferior to that of the male and **hallucinations could stem from the reflux of the menstrual blood to the heart, lungs** etc as the vagina was not yet open by sexual intercourse, hence the common Greek practice of marrying girls off very soon after puberty. He held that intellectual purposes and formal causes guided all natural processes so he arranged the creatures in a graded scale of perfection rising from plants on up to man into a Great Chain of

Being. The **soul was divided into three groups**: a vegetative soul, responsible for reproduction and growth; a sensitive soul, responsible for mobility and sensation; and a rational soul, capable of thought and reflection. He attributed the first only to plants, the first two to animals, and all three to humans. These medical theories of Aristotle have no scientific basis at all and are as hilarious as his geocentric universe, to be contrasted with the Ayurvedic tradition that was 5000 years ahead of its time.

Ancient Greek medicine is synonymous with the name of **Hippocrates** (460- 357 BC) who lived on the island of Cos, travelled extensively, and practiced holistic care; he knew very little anatomy (Figure 9). The Hippocratic Oath is one of the sixty books of the *corpus Hippocraticum* edited 3rd century BC by Alexandrian scholars at the request of Ptolemy, derived from several authors from different periods and Hippocrates merely compiled knowledge assimilated from various sources; Greaves concludes: *"It is impossible to ascribe any particular one to Hippocarates himself"*. Zysk has provided concrete evidence that **historical roots of Ayurveda lie in India**, and not in Greece, as a common heritage of Vedic and Buddhist monks. Greek writers like Arrian and Nearchos, acknowldged the superiority of Vedic physicians over Greeks. Vedic urinanalysis and pulse diagnosis were exceptional and Pythagoras learnt them from Bharat. Hippocrates attributed disease to an imbalance of **four humors** (blood, phlegm, black, and yellow bile) and four bodily conditions (hot, cold, wet and dry) that corresponded to four elements (earth, air, fire, and water). Since there was no Greek philosophical tradition on which to base his theories, Hippocrates must have used knowledge imported from the Vedic traditions through trade and visiting seers, though he speaks of only four elements in place of Ayrurvedic five and does not mention *vata*, *trigunas*, *dhatus*, *ama* and *mala*. The physician Ctesias visited Bharata late 5th century BC.

Hippocrates and others believed that disease outbreaks were cause by *miasma* emerging from dead corpse or rotting matter. So the discovery of germs by Koch 1883 and others met stout resistance and in 1892; a German doctor drank a bear full of cholera bacilli to prove the falsity of the theory. Since breath was the most obvious characteristic of life, **Hippocrates felt that the male sperm was like foam** that transmitted breath inside the womb leading to conception. If the environment inside the womb was not suitable, the sperm would escape as gas. Good internal communication between the respiratory tracts and the uterus was essential for fertility. The **heart** was believed to have a **respiratory function** whereas the **lung** was believed to be related to **blood**

circulation; vessels along the spinal cord were believed to carry the air-rich blood to the bladder, testicles and penis and during this passage the **blood became white sperm** as it reached the testicles. When the testicles are emptied of their sperm, they gradually drain the seminal fluid from the veins immediately above them and the vital spirit from until the whole body is left weak. The right male testicle was believed to give birth to males and left to females; a woman too was believed to have two testicles.

To Hippocrates **menstruation was the absorption of excess blood** from the stomach as her flesh was spongier than that of the boys. Women's breasts were another example of the looseness of the female body as male breasts were firm. Menstruation was believed to have no role in conception but believed to prevent disease in women. So a woman was inferior to man and Aristotle agreed. Hippocrates agreed that the womb was a separate animal inside woman's body, as described by Plato in Timaeus. The **nostrils and the vagina** of a woman were thought to be connected by **one long hollow tube** giving the **womb free passage** from the top to the bottom of the body. To determine whether a woman could conceive, she was made to sit on something strong smelling like garlic; if it could be smelled through her mouth all was well. If not, Hippocrates prescribed applying foul smelling substances to the nostrils while the woman was sitting on a bowl filled with sweet perfumes, thus simultaneously repelling the womb from one end of the body and attracting it to the other. Both Aristotle and Hippocrates thought of a **womb in plural**, as proved by the birth of twins.

Because he could not understand the underlying rationale of humors, Hippocratic treatments consisted of harsh medical practices such as bleeding, purging, vomiting and the administration of highly toxic drugs, to balance the humors by treating symptoms with "opposites." For instance, fever (hot) was believed due to excess blood because patients were flushed, to be balanced by phlebotomy. Greek surgeons used various types of knives, syringes and forceps as surgical tools, almost certainly copied from Sushruta. Hippocrates advocated the use of a few simple herbal drugs - along with fresh air, rest, and proper diet. He frequently accuses air and drinking water of giving rise to disease and suppuration cf *On Airs, Water and Places*. The infectious process was apparently known to him and his semiology details signs and symptoms of various diseases. After the death of Hippocrates, medicine was perfected by his son-in-law Polybus of Cos but many rival schools (Dogmatics, Empirics, Methodists, Pneumatics and Eclectics) sprang up and it was Galen (130-200 CE) who restored the Hippocratic tradition and successfully practiced medicine during the reigns of Antonius, Marcus, Aurelius, Commodus and Pertinax.

Greek men did not approve of female sexual desire, but only as vessels to bear children. Treatment of infertility consisted of opening of the mouth of the womb by a variety of herbal concoctions, ointments, insertion of pessaries into the neck of the womb. Contraception was not much known but the mouth of the womb was blocked by a variety of materials: resin, honey, wax. Abortion was not prohibited but no sure method was available. Childbirth was an occasion of much joy, celebration, temple visits, and could be assisted by violent jerks and medicine if needed.

Archagathus is believed to have introduced the Romans to Greek medicine in 219 BC. Romans used simple remedies that required no professional healer; a *pater familias* **was to doctor his own family**. The immigrant doctors from various corners of the empire brought with them their native knowhow. The Alexandrian School, established 300 BC, was directed by Herophilus of Chalcedon, who corrected Aristotle, placed intelligence in the brain, and connected the nervous system to motion and sensation. **Herophilus and Erasistratus dissected the criminals**, given to them by the king, who were **alive and still breathing**. Herophilus also distinguished between veins and arteries, noting that the latter pulse while the former do not. Erasistratus claimed that the human system of blood vessels was controlled by vacuums, drawing blood across the body. In Erisistratus' physiology, air enters the body, is then drawn by the lungs into the heart, where it is transformed into vital spirit, and is then pumped by the arteries throughout the body. Some of this vital spirit reaches the brain, where it is transformed spirit into animal spirit, which is then distributed by the nerves.

Roman medicine took off only with the arrival of Greeks physicians, either as slaves or freed men. Egyptian physicians were called to Rome as well for specific problems and Roman slaves, racially similar to their masters, had much superior learning when they came from colonies such as Greece. The slaves therefore enjoyed a privileged position and a physician slave was also respected while many female slaves were physicians and active in the government. Cornelius Celsus and Largus in the first millenium CE improvised on Hippocrates and Solanus, knew two abortive methods, but refused to prescribe them; they also paid scant attention to bodily humors. Celsus claimed that dietetics was more important than drugs and surgery. **Life expectancy at birth was 22-25 years**, infant mortality was high but having reached the tenth birthday they could live for an additional 36-38 years. The **population** at the beginning of **first millennium**

CE is believed to number **50-60 million** around the Mediterranean basin; some 10-20% lived in the present day Palestine and Israel.

More than 500 years separated Hippocrates from Claudius **Galenus** (129 – 200 CE), better known as Galen of Pergamum, whose father Nikon, a prosperous architect, was advised in a dream to devote his son to the profession of medicine. He studied at various medical schools including Alexandria, and reached Rome in 162 CE where he was appointed the official doctor of the Imperial Court of Rome. He **dissected thousands of animals** acquiring extensive knowledge of Anatomy which remained unsurpassed until the printed description and illustrations of human dissections by Andreas Vesalius in 1543 CE. Galen's description of the heart, arteries and veins persisted until William Harvey established blood circulation 1628 CE. Galen admitted the four principle humors of Hippocrates and his physiology saw conversion of **food into the Natural Spirit in the liver,** part of which then became the **Vital Spirit after mixing with air in the lung**; after reaching the **brain, the blood was transformed into the Animal Spirit** or breath of the soul. When the testicles were emptied of their sperm, they gradually drain the seminal fluid from the veins immediately above them and the vital spirit from until the whole body was left weak. The right male testicle was believed to give birth to males and left to females; a woman too was believed to have two testicles; good pregnancy meant male child while bad pregnancy meant a female child. Retention during coitus would limit the loss of the vital spirit from which the brain was supposed to form the more elaborate *pneuma* or 'animal spirit'. Sucked into the womb, the life-giving breath 'quickly evaporates' if it does not find a suitable environment. Thick and copious sperm, and not the quantity, were important for procreation though abstinence was favored by Galen. He also advised women to cross their legs after the act in order to keep in this precious sperm. Galen considered that testicles were more important than the heart.

Galen prescribed the use of baths, massage, exercise, defecation, and bloodletting, the latter even on emaciated patients due the theory of humors where the bad had to be replaced by the good. Galen, in contrast to Aristotle, believed that both the male and the female 'seeds' contributed to the formation of the new being. Both Discorides and Galen attributed medicinal properties to stones of various kinds though Galen used few internal remedies except for theriacum and opium because properties of drugs stemmed from four elementary qualities: heat, cold, dampness, dryness. Galen, recommended large doses of drug mixtures - including plant, animal, and mineral ingredients as detailed in *De Materia Medica*.

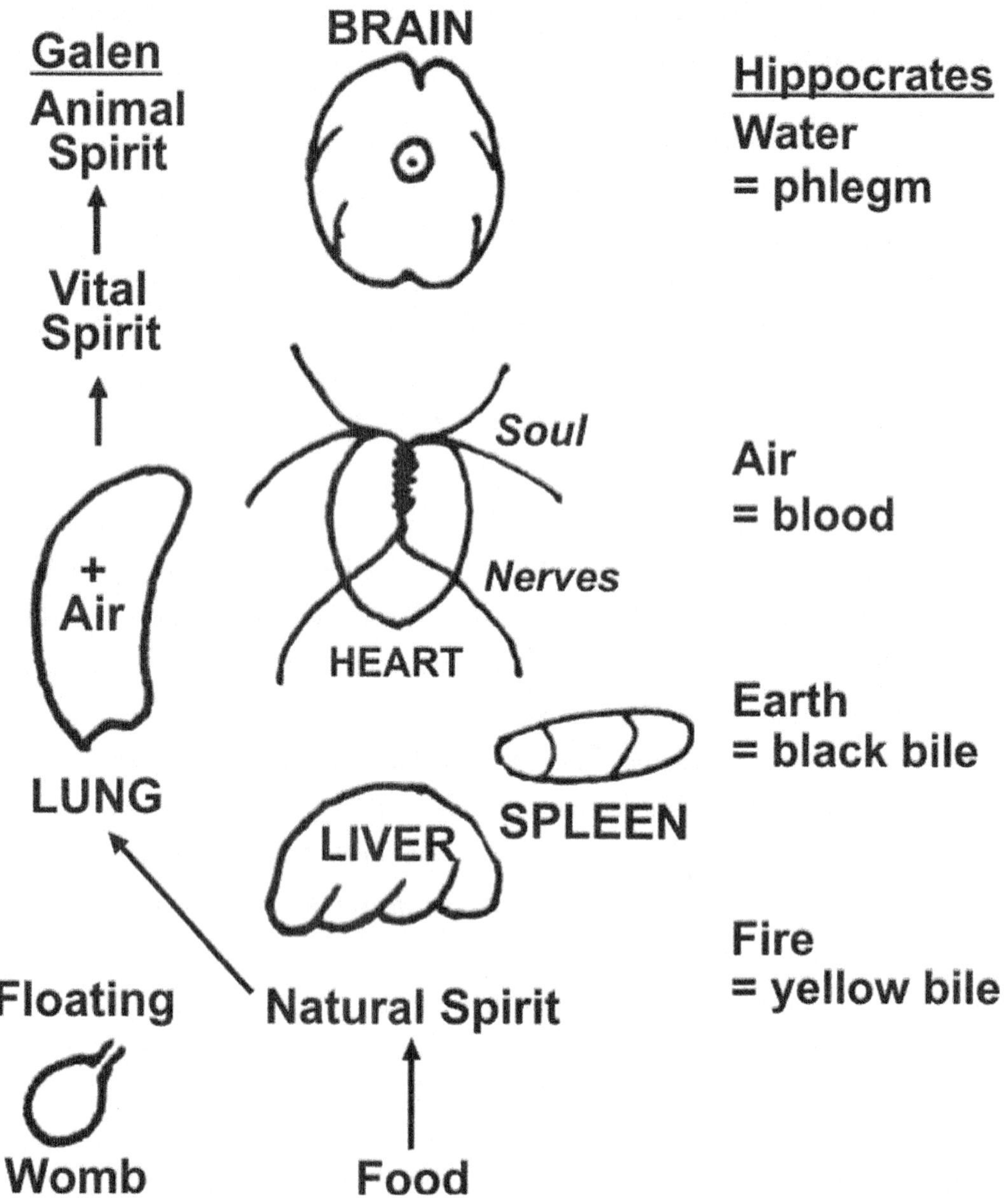

Figure 9. Major preambles of Greek medical theories. Aristotle placed heart as the seat of soul and of the nervous system; he held that semen generated in the brain passed to the penis via heart while in the female some seminal secretion could originate near the diaphragm. He claimed that hair grew out of moisture provided by semen in man's head as the fluid passed through the body to the penis; men were held to be superior to women because the former had more teeth. Both Galen and Plato also suggested the transformation of red blood into white semen either in the brain or in the spinal cord. The four humors of Hippocrates and the three spirits of Galen remain unexplained and the former almost certainly stems from Ayurveda because there is no prior basis for it in the Greek literature. All this is to be contrasted with the advanced physiology and anatomy of Ayurveda, as shown in Figure 10.

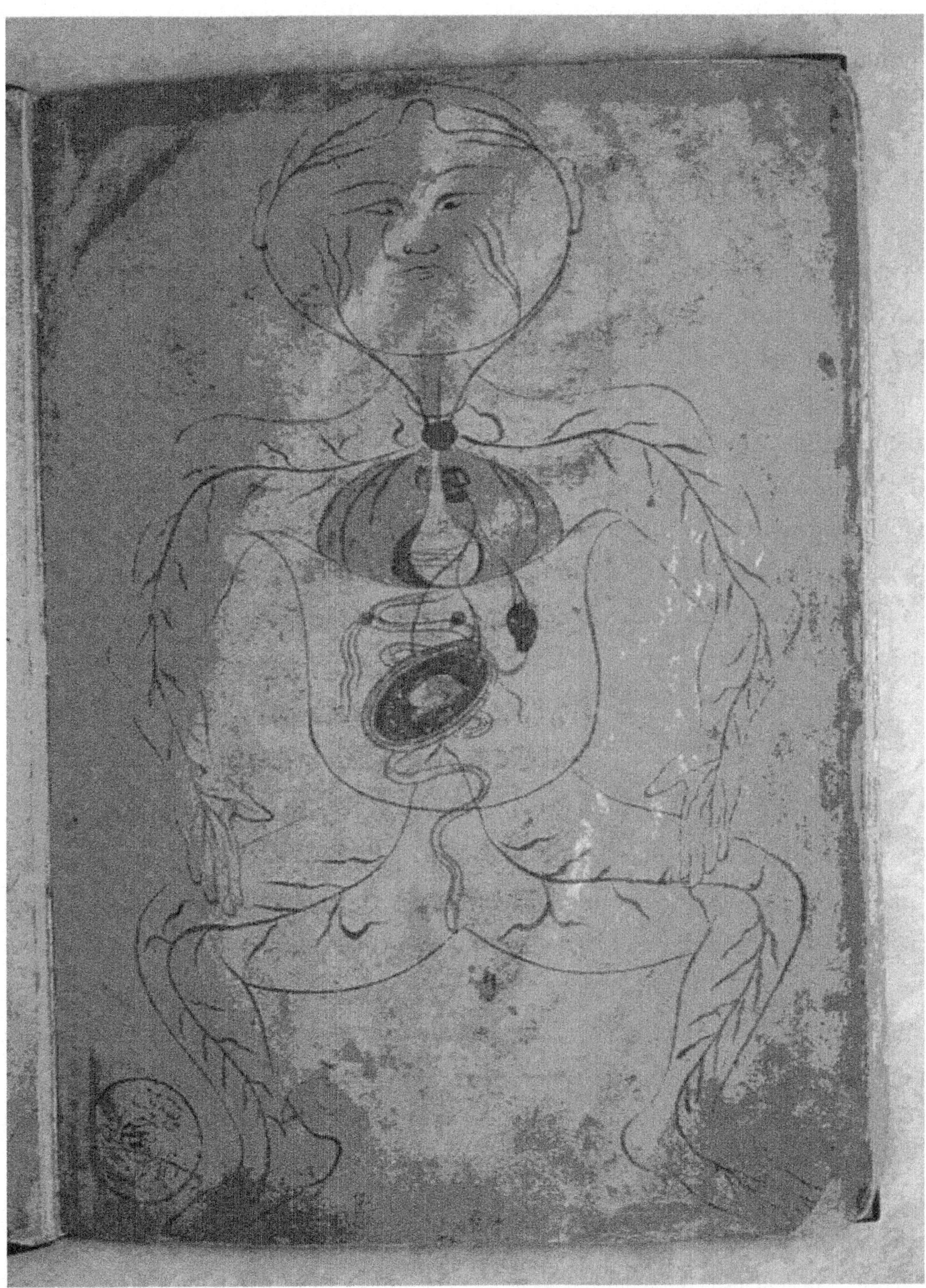

Figure 10. Anatomy and Physiology in Ayurveda. This figure details blood circulation, the digestive tract and the fetus in the uterus; other figures detail various other aspects of human anatomy and physiology (source: a manuscript of the 14th century). These scientific details are to be contrasted with the absurd postulates of Greek medical traditions shown in Figure 9.

Surprisingly little was known about the vagina and Roman girls were married off at 12 or even younger, immediately deflowered, and some became pregnant without their first menstrual period. **Man was supposed to open the way for the flow of the menstrual blood** as vagina was thought to be totally sealed internally although Greeks had pointed out that menstruation occurred in virgin girls. Menses were a type of impure sperm, so the **female was really a castrated male,** believed to occur at the same time in all women, following the cycles of the moon. Once again, conception and pregnancy formed the remedy for all female ailments for a pregnant woman was a healthy woman. Doctors with medical knowledge and access to female patients did not question the philosophic wisdom of Aristotle though Soranus did not agree with it. Amenorrhea was considered a serious disorder that required painful treatments. Highest period of fertility was supposed to follow immediately after menstruation and this misinformation caused a lot of trouble for sexually normal women who did not conceive following coitus after menstrual bleeding. Soranus advised women sex immediately after menstruation if she wanted a child and soon after if she did not wish to conceive. Men wanted very young wives and immediate children due to inheritance laws, lest their inheritance could in part be given away to those relatives who had children. Whereas the Greek marriage contract was between the father of the girl and her future husband, in Rome the marriage contract required the consent of both spouses. After having produced a child, the woman was free to divorce and to terminate future pregnancy.

Soranus compared mother to the seedbed that had to be planted and men had complete control over her body. Soranus viewed menstruation as harmful yet a necessary antecedent to pregnancy. **Uterine amulets** were common in the Roman Empire, and were used to retain menses during gestation for nourishing the uterus. At the time of delivery, a child was examined for physical defects and the umbilical cord was cut only if the child was worth raising, and if the prospective father took the baby boy in his arms as part of his family; girls were not picked up in this manner. The mother had no say in the matter and it is not clear what happened to the **imperfect child** though they **were abandoned and left to die.** The child's body was molded by nurses by regular massage, baths, nose lift, rounding off of heads, etc until the age of 6 or 7. As penis was to be later on seen by dozens of men everyday at the baths and/or gymnasium, the size and shape were corrected by scrotum massage and gentle stretching of the foreskin over the glans. **Mother's milk (colostrum)** was held to be too heavy for the baby to digest; **and harmful for 20 days (Soranus) or 40 days (Mnesitheus)** until the mother recovered for the production of good quality of milk. The fact that the wet nurse herself was a mother did not enter into consideration and her child would be fed on cereal or whatever. The nurse had to be selected carefully for her breast shape, softness, texture, health, and several nurses per child were recommended. After six months, the baby was exposed to wine, honey, cereal, bread but water as such was discouraged. Tutors were appointed at the age of six or seven and the appearance of pubic hair and ejaculation were celebrated by the whole household.

Child sacrifice, group sexual orgies, incest, and castration, were practiced freely. Child sacrifice could be part of the initiation ceremony, sometimes practiced publicly, where the child covered in dough was put on a table, slaughtered by the neophyte, and the onlookers would then **dip bread in the child's blood and eat** it. According to Tertullian, **child sacrifices** were public **affairs** in **North Africa** until first century CE, paid for and organized by the community, and the **sexual organs of a priest were adored, as was the head of an ass.** Castration could lead a man to the innocence of a child and thus a perfect victim for Satan; it could also transform his *pneuma* into something entirely psychic as there could be no more loss of vital seed and was thus guaranteed eternal life. In the **2ⁿᵈ century CE, children were still thrown from the top of the temple of Atargatis, by parents who joked as they did so.** Sacred prostitution in the worship of Baal was prevalent at this time and some men renounced fertility by surgical removal of testicles but they did not renounce sexuality.

Discussion of virginity became something of a fashion during the 4ᵗʰ century, bishops preaching it to young girls of aristocratic birth to dissuade them from accepting a husband. Another body of treatises dealt with the manner in which **young boys would be sent to monk's care** to escape being sexually initiated, generally at the age of ten in Roman Africa. Men went to the monastic life in the deserts of Egypt to avoid temptation of seeing women and thus love God only by living on roots, grains, and plants. Visiting young boys, more than women, tempted the monks and **sexual violations** took place. **The monks did not have to atone for the sexual act** but tried to subdue the body by fasting. Masturbation was also talked about and wet dreams were written off as natural events for which men were not responsible. Monks were forbidden to lock their cell doors in an attempt to prevent masturbation. Some monks like Antony and Theonas blamed the Devil for wet dreams and ejaculations. Carnal relationships between monks grew in Monasteries. Until a thousand years ago, popular birth control methods in the Western world included spitting into the mouth of a frog, eating bees and wearing the testicles of a weasel. In Cordoba, Spain, supposed to be at the cutting edge of science and medicine, women were told to leap up and down vigorously after sex, and then jump backwards nine times, to avoid conception. (International Herald Tribune 10 May 2010).

Apollonius of Tyana came to Bharata from Greece and took back much of the knowledge with him. During the middle Ages and the Renaissance, the spice trade brought many Ayurveda herbs to Europe. The alchemical tradition from Europe to China was based in Ayurveda during this same period as it was heavily proscribed by the Church in Europe. Hildegard of Binger (12th CE Germany) used many Ayurvedic herbs like the long pepper (pippali), gems and minerals. Ficino mentions many Ayurvedic herbs (Triphala, aloe, saffron, cinnamon and cloves) and formulae in his work: *The Book of Life*. In Asclepius one finds the infiltration of the eastern tradition into archaic Greece. Wandering seers from Vratyas, Jains and Ajivika traditions had found all the way to Greece via Persia. Greek writers Arrian and Nearchos acknowledged the superiority of Hindu physicians over those from Greece. In fact, the **medical tradition assigned to the Hippocrates in Greece was an idea invented primarily by the British to assert white racial superiority**. Indeed, there was no written source anywhere in the world for the development of medical discipline, in contrast to the vast Vedic literature.

Persian. Persian classics like Avesta and the Gathas consist of hymns thought to have been composed by Zarathushtra (Zoroaster) himself, and dated linguistically to around 1000 BC. The various *Yashts* are in Younger Avestan and thought to date to the Achaemenid era (559–330 BC). The medical history of ancient Persia can be divided into **three distinct periods**. The *Visprad* and *Vendidad*, which are also in Younger Avestan, were probably composed even later. The word *Zend* or *Zand*, literally meaning "interpretation", refers to late Middle Persian era. The sixth book of Zend-Avesta contains some of the earliest records of history of ancient Iranian medicine. In a passage of the Vendidad (Given against the Demons), one of the surviving texts of the Zendavesta, three kinds of medicine were distinguished: medicine by the knife (surgery), medicine by herbs, and medicine by divine words. Although the Avesta mentions several physicians, the most notable of Persia's ancient physicians were to emerge later, namely: Mani, Roozbeh, and Bozorgmehr. The second era begins with the Achaemenid dynasty (559-330 BC), until the reign of Darius I. The third epoch covers the era of what is known as Pahlavi literature (300 BC – 900 CE) where the entire subject of medicine was incorporated in the encyclopedic work of Dinkart which lists some 4333 diseases. The medicine of the Medes and the Persians somewhat resembled that of the Chaldeans. Vendidad says that Ahriman created by his evil eye 99,999 diseases in the form of demons, and mentions a code for purification – literally *"The law against demons"*. When Ormuzd appealed for aid to *Aryaman*, a god of heavenly light mentioned in the *Vedas*, *Aryaman* destroyed the diseases by reciting the holy word. Ormuzd also took 10,000 healing herbs and brought them to Thrita, an ancient sage and *Vedic* personage, who also received the knife from Kshathra-Vairya, Lord of the metals. Egyptian influence also permeated Persia where Avesta describes various diseases to be treated with incantations. The Persian science was interrupted by the Arab invasion (630 CE). To save the books from the Arab carnage, many Pahlavi writings were translated into the Arabic, and Iran produced physicians and scientists like Avicenna and Raz, and mathematicians as Kharazmi and Khayyam, who systematically expanded the Greek, Indian, and Persian medical heritage.

Arabic and European Middle Ages

After Galen, medicine in Europe (200 to 1500 CE) was forgotten as Medical diplomas did not exist in either the Empire or the Republican Rome where 1000 or more male and female tutelary powers presided over all diseases and needs. The Alexandrian school of medicine declined with the rise of Christianity. The medicine in the Old Testament betrays both Egyptian and Babylonian influence; **divination** was practiced widely as disease stemmed from a chemistry of **stars, sorcery and demoniacal influences**. Anyone could practice the art without qualification and made the medicines themselves based upon their own experience. Everywhere during the Middle Ages, learning was the handmaiden of Theology; disease was the **wrath of gods** and had to be cured by clemency of gods. Free thinking and inquiry were not allowed in the fixed theological setting of the Semites and Christians. Greeks learned from India and Iran but they were destroyed by Romans and Christians, more so after the Roman Emperor was converted to Christianity. Philosophy, science, mathematics, medicine etc were largely eliminated from Europe by the 6th century CE. European universities basically copied religious texts and edited it to their taste but did not understand the text. Medicine meant blessing of the priests as Christians enforced that **hygiene should be abandoned** because Jesus had said ***"but to eat with unwashen hands defileth not the man"***, in contrast to the Vedic practice dating back to the ISC. Segregation was unknown, the toilet pot was kept inside the house until after WW II and **hands or bottom were never washed** though rags were used. Diet consisted of barley gruel with vegetables and bread, occasional cheese and fruit. Average **life span was 35** and over one half children died before five during the Dark Ages. Helplessness meant prayer was the only answer just like as *Bhakti* movement in India under Muslim rule. It was believed that all useful knowledge had already been written in the Bible so Galileo was persecuted and Copernicus laughed at for their heliocentric universe. Chaucer's Canterbury tales make fun of an astrologer for studying moon and stars which were God's private affairs.

Attraction and desire to other people's bodies, or *porneia*, was seen by thinkers as obstructing, obsessing, and disturbing reason and the freedom of mind. Politicians, medical writers, and scholars all agreed that desire reflected an enslaved mind which should not be allowed to intrude into intellectual or political life. Intellectual castration, invented and preached by the Jewish, spread to Greek and Roman empires. Thus, Christians reduced **sex and fertility as stumbling blocks to reunion with God**. The idea that **disease is a consequence of evil conduct** was so prominent in Europe that, when Jenner discovered smallpox vaccination, debates raged all over Europe whether the disease should be suffered as a punishment, or whether it was acceptable to prevent recurrence. Muslim Mid East, too, debated whether to cure lethal diseases such as plague. It was only in the 18th century that Enlightenment finally abandoned the Biblical idea that mental illness was caused by diabolical possessions. AIDS spread is now being used by religious fundamentalists as divine punishment.

The uses of plants for medicine and other purposes changed little in early medieval Europe. Many Greek and Roman writings on medicine, as on other subjects, were preserved by hand copying of manuscripts in monasteries. The monasteries thus tended to become local centers of medical knowledge, and their herb gardens provided the raw materials for simple treatment of common disorders. At the same time, folk medicine at home and in villages continued uninterrupted, supporting numerous wandering and settled herbalists. Among these were the "wise-women," who prescribed herbal remedies often along with spells and enchantments. However, in the late Middle Ages, women knowledgeable in herb lore became the targets of the witch hunt hysteria. One of the most famous women in the herbal tradition was Hildegard of Bingen, a twelfth century Benedictine nun, who wrote a medical text called *Causes and Cures*.

Arab medical tradition starts with the translations they made from Greek, Latin, Babylonian and Vedic-Buddhist-Jain texts so **Ayurveda became well known to the Arab world as early as 700 CE.** Avicenna (980-1036 CE) compiled a vast encyclopedia which formed the standard textbook of medicine for the Latin west until the 17th century CE. As a result, Yunani medicine was born in Baghdad during the 8th century 'from the ashes of the Alexandrian library' which contained medical texts from Greece and Bharata. Charaka Samhita was translated from Sanskrit to Persian and from Persian into Arabic; the name *sharaka indianus* can be found in the Latin translation of Rhazes (68 CE). Madhava was translated around 850 CE by al-Tabari and reached Europe soon after. Sushruta samhita was translated into Arabic 800 CE under the title *Kitabshahshun-al-hindi*. He heavily borrowed many Vedic-Buddhist medical traditions and his *Canon of Medicine* lists 800 tested drugs, plants and minerals.

Abulcasis of Cordoba (936-1013 CE) authored *The Book of Simples*, an important source for later European herbals, while Ibn al-Baitar of Malaga (1197-1248 CE) compiled the *Corpus of Simples*, which introduced 200 new healing herbs, including tamarind, aconite, and nux vomica. Other books were written by Abu-Rayhan Biruni in the 11th century and Ibn Zuhr (Avenzoar) in the 12th centuryCE. The 15th-17th, centuries were the great age of herbals, many of them available for the first time in English and other languages other than Latin or Greek. The first herbal to be published in English was the anonymous *Grete Herball* in 1526 CE, followed by the *General History of Plants* (1597 CE) by John Gerard, and *The English Physician Enlarged* by Nicholas Culpeper (1653 CE). Gerard's text was basically a pirated translation of a book by the Belgian herbalist Dodoens and his illustrations came from a German botanical work. Culpeper's blend of traditional medicine with astrology, magic, and folklore was ridiculed by the physicians of his day yet his book - like Gerard's and other herbals - enjoyed phenomenal popularity. The Age of Exploration and the Columbian Exchange introduced new medicinal plants to Europe. The *Badianus Manuscript* was an illustrated Aztec herbal translated into Latin in the 16th century CE.

Medical schools known as Bimaristan began to appear from the 9th century CE in the medieval Islamic world, which was generally more advanced than medieval Europe at the time. Baghdad became as important center for Arab herbalism between 800 and 1400 CE. Al-Dinawari described more than 637 plant drugs in the 9th century, and Ibn al-Baitar in the 13th century described more than 1,400 different plants, foods and drugs, over 300 of which were his own original discoveries. The experimental scientific method was introduced into the field of *materia medica* in the 13ᵗʰ century by the Andalusian-Arab botanist Abu al-Abbas al-Nabati, the teacher of Ibn al-Baitar. Al-Nabati introduced empirical techniques in the testing, description and identification of numerous specimens of *materia medica*, and he separated unverified reports from those supported by actual tests and observations, all of which led to the development of pharmacology. The origins of clinical pharmacology also date back to Avicenna's *The Canon of Medicine*, Peter of Spain's *Commentary on Isaac*, and John of St Amand's *Commentary on the Antedotary of Nicholas*. In particular, the *Canon* introduced clinical trials, randomized controlled trials, and efficacy tests.

The story of the founding of European Universities goes no farther than the Enlightenment in the 13ᵗʰ century at Bologna and Paris, just at the time when Nalanda in India was being destroyed by the Muslims. Arnold of Villanova at Montpellier followed Arabic medical traditions and did not make much contribution of his own. He was constantly in trouble with the Church as his writings were condemned to be heretical. Henri de Mandeville was also dominated by the Arabs and the idea of humors, astrology, divination, charms and so forth continued although conflicting with the church view of the Divine Will. **Arabic texts now formed the staple curriculum and revived Greek traditions while Hindus were forgotten**. Padua became the center of Anatomy around 1600 CE and Harvey studied there as well. The hygiene in European Middle Ages was below the level in the Roman Empire. Until the middle of the sixteenth century, physiology and anatomy remained much the same as taught by Galen who respected the Aristotelian tradition of heart as the nerve center. Galenic teachings began to be questioned at the end of the Middle Ages and with the founding of the universities where Arabic texts formed the staple curriculum and revived Greek traditions while **Hindus were forgotten. The first recorded public dissection of the human body** was **performed in Bologna ca 1315** by Mondino de'Liuzzi (1270-1326 CE) and two theaters of dissection were established, one each in Venice (1552 CE) and Montpellier (1556 CE) although Rabelais had dissected in Montpellier in 1532 CE. Anatomy thereafter became the queen of sciences for the next three centuries and greatly helped surgical techniques. Andreas Vesalius (1514-1564 CE) of Belgium was a great anatomist who became a professor of anatomy and surgery in Padua. Contagious nature of diseases was also evident but the theories of Galen led to skepticism.

Chemistry revolutionized healing after **Paracelsus** (1493-1541 CE) of Switzerland, also known as the Father of Modern Western Medicine, introduced chemicals to treat syphilis; he also came up with the idea that *homunculi* could be made by placing human sperm plus horse dung into retort and baking it for 40 days. Leeuwenhoek (1632-1723 CE) described '*animalcules*' which were complete minuscule human beings with their own sex organs who then had their 'animalcules' *ad infinitum*. Paracelsus laid the foundation of modern chemical physiology but he **borrowed heavily from Ayurveda.** He was the first to declare that, if given in small doses, "*What makes a man ill also cures him,*" an anticipation of Homeopathy. It is not surprising that Paracelsus was called a magician because at the time **science and magic were still entwined**; the study of one meant the study of the other, therefore sanctioned by the Church. He believed in natural magic (power) in all things "*Power that comes direct from God*". Included in Paracelsus' belief in natural power was astrology. He held that the stars and planets influenced life and matter. One of his most significant beliefs was that man's soul and body were inseparable:

> "*Man is not body. The heart, the spirit, is man. And this spirit is an entire star, out of which, he is built. If therefore a man is perfect in his heart, nothing in the whole light of Nature is hidden from him.*"

For Descartes, **embryogenesis was like the fermentation** of a particle containing fluid that is acted upon by mechanical forces: heat and movement; this is philosophy not science or medicine. Harvey proposed that **conception was akin to a contagion** communicated to the womb by the semen. It was unthinkable that conception could result from the admixture of two unorganized fluids, in **contrast to Ayurveda** where heredity and genetics were already described (chapter 6). Chemical embryology had to wait the idea of signals proposed by Hans Spenann (1869-1941 CE) for which a Nobel Prize was awarded to him. First caesarian sections were performed in Europe only in the late 18th early 19th century CE, in contrast to the Ayurvedic tradition of 1000 BC.

Physical diagnosis was introduced only at the end of the nineteenth century when **Hospital medicine evolved in France 1789-1848 CE**, in contrast to the age old traditions of Ayurveda back to 1000 BC or more (chapter 9). The emphasis was now laid on inspection, palpation, percussion, stethoscope (Laennec), and *post mortum* dissection. X-rays entered the scene towards the end of the 19th century. Because women were regarded as property, physicians could not look at them and a thick screen sometimes separated the woman from the physician. The vaginal speculum, although practiced freely in Europe, was adamantly rejected in North America as outrageously immoral. X-ray introduced a dilemma as now a woman could be unveiled and a New Jersey congressman tried to introduce a law barring it. The Credit for blood pressure measurement goes to Stephen Hales (1677-1761 CE). Transfusion of lamb's blood into the humans were performed in 1667 CE in London and in Paris in 1668 CE but forbidden by the courts when the recipient died. Medieval religious theocracy, philosophy, and general antipathy towards scientific investigation, stifled new approaches and ideas.

Urine inspection was practiced as of the 12th century CE although a document from the 6th century already says that the urine *"tells a skilled physician the whole history of his patient's disease"*. Stool examination was recorded for the first time by Pierre Bourdelot, private physician to the Duke of Bourbon (1692-1740 CE). Public health movement began only in the 19th century, in contrast to the cleanliness of the ISC 3000 BC, and Jenner's paper on inoculation was refused by the Royal Society. During the cholera epidemic of 1832 CE bureaucrats looked for indiscrimating smell in the sewers though the cholera organism was described by Filipo Pacini (1812-1883 CE). During Renaissance, calculus from the indigestible materials in the stomachs of some animals (gazelles, goats, llamas) were used to treat melancholia and toxic states. Also used were the Egyptiam mummy and the unicorn's horn. Enemas were immensely used and King Louis XIV is said to have received some 2000 of them, sometimes three or four a day. Psychiatry did not come of age before the 19th century in Europe whereas psychoanalysis was recognized only in the 20th century Europe, again in contrast to the Ayurvedic tradition of 1000 BC or earlier.

Babylonian.

The cuneiform texts reveal the lowest form of medicine and Chaldeans contributed absolutely nothing to it because demons caused disease. Here prayers, charms and offerings formed the only cure. The patients were therefore put on public squares in the hope that passers by would come wih some suggestion. Assyrian literature under Ashurbanipal (669-626 BC) recounted mythological poems of Sumerians e.g. Poem of Creation (Enuna Eliah) and Gilgamesh; other works imitated the ancient Sumerian or Accadian Hymns to Gods, incantations, ritual writings, genealogies of kings, victories and defeats. The first text book on medicine is the *Diagnostic Handbook*, written by the physician Esagil-kin-apli of Borsippa, during the reign of the Babylonian king Adad-apla-iddina (1069-1046 BC). As with the ancient Egyptian medicine, the Babylonians followed diagnosis, prognosis, physical examination, prescriptions, therapy and etiology, using empiricism, logic and rationality. Therapy included bandages, creams, pills and exorcism.

Chinese.

The Yellow river valley was home to an infinite number of ethnic groups and languages but, in the Chinese version, history begins with three semi-mystical and legendary individuals who taught civilization around 2800-2600 BC: Fu Hsi, the inventor of writing, hunting, trapping, and fishing; Shen Nung, the inventor of agriculture and mercantilism, and the Yellow Emperor who invented government and Taoist philosophy but all of this is dismissed by Western historians. The Cultural Heroes were followed by the Three Sage Kings, Yao (around 2350 BC), Shun (around 2250 BC), and Yu (rule began in 2205 BC). The Five Classics of China go no farther back than the first half of the 1st millennium BC and were used by Confucianism as the basis for their studies *I-ching* The Book of Changes (divination); *Shu-ching* The book of Documents (Chou history); *Shih-ching* The Book of Odes (ancient songs and poems); The Book of Rites (society, government, ceremonial rites); The Book of Spring/Autumn Annals (diplomatic relations, alliances and military actions, births and deaths of the ruling families). In the I Ching and other Chinese literary and philosophical classics, general principles of health and healing are mentioned but the first Chinese herbal book, the *Shennong Bencao Jing*, was compiled only during the Han Dynasty (206-222 BC). It lists 365 medicinal plants and their uses, including *ma-Huang*, a shrub that introduced ephedrine to modern medicine but almost half of the botanical sources listed here are also described in earlier texts of Ayurveda. Succeeding generations expanded on the *Shennong Bencao Jing*, as in the *Yaoxing Lun* (Treatise on the Nature of Medicinal Herbs), a 7th century CE Tang Dynasty treatise on herbal medicine.

The Traditional Chinese medicine (TCM) as of 1900 BC was diverse and catered to local demands. It borrowed heavily from Taoism, Buddhism, Neo-Confucianism and Ayurveda but remained static until the modern era. The human body was at the center of the universe and governed by *qi*, loosely translated as the 'Life Force', consisting of water, earth, metal, wood and fire. The *qi* is made up of the *Yin* and *Yang* (or 'opposites') - the feminine and masculine principles - that are balanced by the four bodily humors (*qi*, blood, moisture and essence) and internal organ systems (*zang fu*); any imbalance in *qi* led to disease. The TCM model of the body is based on the meridian system of Ayurveda where 107 *marmas* in Sushruta Samhita correspond with the topographical points of the inner vital organs, but their significance was lost due to wrong interpretations and translations of Sanskrit texts. Earlier, it was thought that Vedic *dhamanis* and the *siras* represent arteries and veins but in reality these are channels and meridians that control the vital energy flow. Thus, the *marmas* were important groups of *siras* and not just tissues to be saved during surgical operations. Consequently, *marmas* **and meridians of** *Sushruta Samhita* **are the basis of Chinese acupuncture** (Dr. Binod Kumar Joshi et al, Motilal Banarasidas, in press). Although the Semites, Egypt, Tao, and Mesopotamia, have all been credited with similar ideas, the tradition never developed later in any of these locations. In particular, Tao believed in forcing the semen up the spine to the brain but Han texts profess a similar doctrine.

Egyptian

The Egyptian literature 2600 - 2200 BC included funerary texts, epistles and letters, religious hymns and poems, and commemorative autobiographical texts recounting the careers of prominent administrative officials. It records the laments of Isis over the corpse of Osiris, some fiction, adventure, mythology etc but narrative works appear only during the Middle Kingdom (2100 - 1700 BC). Isis and Osiris invented medicine in Egyptian mythology and Isis taught it to her son Horus, as per the four Egyptian payrus texts of 2000 BC. Anatomy is described in 4000 BC texts ascribed to Athothis, the son and successor of Menes who had founded the first dynasty. A book of proverbs details the teachings of Amenemope (1077 - 943 BC) which appears to have influenced the Hebrew book of Proverbs. Imhotep in the 3rd dynasty (2667 - 2648 BC), is credited as the original author of the papyrus text, and founder of ancient Egyptian medicine. In 1822, the Rosetta stone finally allowed the translation of ancient Egyptian hieroglyphic inscriptions on the Ebers papyrus, the Edwin Smith Papyrus, the Hearst Papyrus, and others dating back as far as 3000 BC. The Edwin Smith Papyrus (ca1600 BC) is a textbook on surgery and details anatomical observations and the examination, diagnosis, treatment, and prognosis of numerous ailments. The Ebers papyrus (ca 1550 BC) is full of incantations and foul applications to turn away disease-causing demons.

During the Pharaohs, Theophrastus, Galen and Dioscorides frequently quote prescriptions that they learnt at the temple of Aesculapius at Memphis. Egyptian physicians could treat eye afflictions 500 years before the Christian era, **(but much later than Vedic practice),** used anesthetics, had devised some semeiology and pathology and medical schools were founded from the very first dynasty. The earliest known surgery was performed in Egypt around 2750 BC. From 3300 BC to 523 BC, Egyptian medicine included simple, non-invasive surgery, setting of bones and an extensive set of pharmacopoeia. Egyptian physicians were aware of the existence of the pulse and of a connection between pulse and heart. Egyptian theory linked bone marrow, especially in the spine, with male sperm, based on an earlier Greek version of the fifth century, according to Hippo.

The author of the Smith Papyrus even had a vague idea of a cardiac system, although not of blood circulation and he was unable, or deemed it unimportant, to distinguish between blood vessels, tendons, and nerves. They developed their theory of "channels" that carried air, water and blood to the body by analogies with the River Nile; if it became blocked, crops became unhealthy and they applied this principle to the body: If a person was unwell, they would use laxatives to unblock the "channels". There were inspectors of doctors, overseers and chief doctors. Known ancient Egyptian specialists are ophthalmologist, gastroenterologist, proctologist, dentist, "doctor who supervises butchers" and an unspecified "inspector of liquids". The relationship between Egyptian and Ayurvedic traditions remains to be elucidated.

The Americas.

Aztecs possessed a vast knowledge of medicinal plants and Montezuma I owned extensive Botanical gardens. Friars, who accompanied the Spanish, acknowledged that **Aztec physicians could cure chronic diseases that resisted European therapy**. In contrast to the use of boiling oil or of red hot iron to control bleeding, the Aztecs were using the extracts of the plant *Commelina pallida* which is now known to promote coagulation and vascular constriction. Aztecs were also good at treating burns, bites, provoking uterine contractions, subduing pain with *Argemone grandiflora* which is similar to opium, inflammation by *Disoscorea*; quinine was taken to Europe by the Jesuits, along with ephedra, digitalis, etc. British physician Thomas Sydenham (1624-1689 CE) used Peruvian bark to cure malaria and questioned the Hippocratic humors. Peruvians made use of the antiseptic properties of tree resins, and used anesthetics. Nevertheless, the Spanish criticized Aztecs for not compounding plant extracts and forgetting blood letting whose 'curative' virtues could be sworn by every self-respecting European physician of the 16th century CE. Some 70% of contemporary Western pharmacopeia stems from the knowledge in the Americas.

Allopathy. The term "allopathy" was invented by the German physician Samuel Hahnemann (1755-1843 CE) by joining *allos* "opposite" and *pathos* " to replace the *"law of similia"* that treated "like with like,". Hahnemann had abandoned medical practice because of his inability to heal his patients by the methods of his era. The label "allopath" was considered highly derisive by regular medicine. A 1902 CE book, intended for new medical graduates, reveals just how vehemently Medical Doctors once opposed and resented the label:

> *"Allopath is a false nickname not chosen by regular physicians at all, but cunningly coined, and put in wicked use against us…The term Allopathy applied to regular medicine is both untrue and offensive and is no more accepted by us than the term "Heretics" is accepted by the Protestants, or "Niggers" by the Blacks".*

An alternate definition of allopathy would be: *"a system of medical practice making use of all measures proved of value in treatment of disease"*. This definition accurately describes modern, science-based medicine, but is inconsistent with its root words "allos" and "pathos." The duplicity of the term aids those who wish to misrepresent medicine as ideologically allopathic (i.e., symptom suppression). Although medicine never accepted the label of allopathy, nonmedical practitioners such as chiropractors, homeopaths, and naturopaths regularly misrepresent physicians as "allopaths." This is usually done in order to underline conflicting philosophies, rather than ideology versus science. Opponents claim that they treat the underlying causes of disease, while MDs treat only the symptoms. Further, they claim that medicine suppresses the symptoms, thus interfering with the body's inherent healing processes.

Chiropractics appreciated the workings of:

> *"Universal Intelligence (God); the function of Innate Intelligence (Soul, Spirit or Spark of Life) within each; and the fundamental causes of interference to the planned expression of that Innate Intelligence in the form of Mental, Chemical and/or Mechanical Stresses, which create the structural distortions that interfere with nerve supply…Our way is to research the mystery and beauty of the life force, in which we have faith. Our power and our responsibility is to bring the life force into the light."*

Chiropractic manipulative therapy's main aim is the symptomatic relief from back pain.

Homeopathy. In the late 1700s, Samuel Hahnemann, a physician, chemist, and linguist in Germany, proposed a new approach to treating illness. At that time the most common medical treatments were harsh, such as bloodletting, purging, blistering, and the use of sulfur and mercury. Hahnemann was interested in developing a less-threatening approach to medicine. While translating an herbal text, he read about a treatment (cinchona bark) used to cure malaria. He took some cinchona bark and observed that, as a healthy person, he developed symptoms that were very similar to malaria symptoms. This led Hahnemann to consider that a substance may create symptoms that it can also relieve or the *"similia principle"* or *"like cures like"*. The similia principle goes back to Hippocrates who noted that recurrent vomiting could be treated with an emetic (such as ipecacuanha) that would be expected to make it worse. The *"like cures like"* is body's attempt to heal itself e.g. fever can develop as a result of an immune response to an infection, and a cough helps eliminate mucus. Medication may thus be given to support this self-healing response. Homeopathy has always been symptomatic, based upon a process called "proving" which identifies prospective remedies by matching the symptoms they produce in high dosages with the symptoms reported by a patient.

Hahnemann added two additional elements to homeopathy. First, "Potentiation," holds that systematically diluting a substance, with vigorous shaking at each step of dilution, makes the remedy more, not less, effective by extracting the vital essence of the substance. If dilution is continued to a point where the substance's molecules are gone, the mere "memory" of them on the surrounding water molecules may still be therapeutic. Second, treatment should be selected based upon a total picture of an individual and not solely upon symptoms of a disease; emotions, mental states, lifestyle, nutrition, and other aspects should also be considered. Thus, different people with the same symptoms may receive different homeopathic remedies.

Hans Burch Gram, a Boston-born doctor, studied homeopathy in Europe and introduced it to the United States in 1825 CE. European immigrants trained in homeopathy also made the treatment increasingly available in America. The first homeopathic medical college was established in Allentown, Pennsylvania in 1835 CE, and by the 20th century there were 20 homeopathic medical colleges and more than 100 homeopathic hospitals. The medical advances of the late 19th and early 20th centuries, such as the recognition of the mechanisms of disease, Pasteur's germ theory, antiseptic techniques, ether anesthesia, all had a negative effect on homeopathy. Most homeopathic medical schools closed down, and by the 1930s the remainder had converted to conventional medical schools. In the 1960s, homeopathy's popularity began to revive in the United States. According to a 1999 survey, over 6 million Americans had used homeopathy in the preceding 12 months. The World Health Organization noted in 1994 that homeopathy was integrated into the national health care systems of numerous countries, including Germany, the United Kingdom, India, Pakistan, Sri Lanka, and Mexico.

Naturopathy. Naturopaths claim to be the inheritors of the Hippocratic tradition, and pay lip service to the *Vis Medicatrix Naturae,* but their belief in the "life force" reveals that they do not understand the most important point of Hippocrates's revolutionary proposition that the healing power of nature was not a supernatural force. Naturopathy is eclectic, but none of its nonstandard medical modalities is truly aimed at causation.

Vitalism. A number of healing systems are rooted in *vitalism*:

> "*A doctrine that the functions of a living organism are due to a vital principle distinct from physicochemical forces*" or, "*the theory that biological activities are directed by a supernatural force which denotes a paranormal life force.*"

Vitalists are not just nonscientific, they are *antiscientific* because they abhor reductionism (versus holism) of science, the materialism (versus etherealism) of science, and the mechanistic (versus mystical) processes of science. They prefer subjective experience to objective testing, and place intuitiveness above reason and logic. Vitalism is a powerful motivating force because it is inextricably linked to the concept of an immortal human soul - a piece of the Divine that is the essence of existence. This connects vitalism to religious ideologies and explains why Sarton stated that the vitalist point of view dodges every blow and reappears under a new form.

17.

Perspectives

Buddha, along with Mahavira, rebelled against the traditional practices from which the Vedic society never recovered. Sacrifices were replaced by consciousness and quietitude of the mind, thus ending the Brahmin monopoly. A new set of gurus now came up to instill the ideas of **ahimsa, asteya, satya, saucha and atmanigrah** while reincarnation, transmigration and **avatars** gained ground. Brahmanism evolved into Hinduism and *Bhakti* became the way to God by worshipping personal images along with natural objects. Practically nothing was left of the sacred gardens called *tapovans* where elite Brahmins presided over elaborate Vedic sacrifices and rituals. The principles of Kapila and Patanjali found an honorable place in the society as well but Swamis and Goswamis became masters of their own self. **Submission, tolerance and non-violence replaced Vedic ambitions**. The combined effect of Buddhism and Jainism gave birth to Vaishnavism but neo-Brahmanism began to emerge in the south perhaps because of the migration of Egyptian and Iranian Brahmins to India. They aligned themselves with the local rulers to exploit the serfs and the untouchables while Vedic laws began to emerge in a new garb of rituals, pilgrimages, holy days and nights, arts, grammar and mathematics. Ayurveda itself changed to reflect new realities. Animal products were abandoned to such an extent that Ayruveda has now become almost synonymous with herbal medicine though minerals are used as well. Today, people refuse to believe that Ayrurveda used products of animal origin, much like they refuse to believe that our Vedic ancestors consumed meat, and that ancient Bharata was a land of sexual freedom.

The appearance of two new universal religions was to change events the likes of which the world had never witnessed before. Jesus had travelled widely and had absorbed the major spiritual knowledge available at that time. He was a fully accomplished *advaita jnana yogi*, when he resusitated the ancient Vedic ideation: ***"I and my father are One"***, ***"I am in Ye, you are in me"***, ***"I am He"*** which is essentially the same as *tat tvam asi*. When he said *"The Truth will make you free"*, no one could understand him; he therefore had to limit himself to *yama, niyama* and *bhakti* as Vedanta was never meant for the masses. Thomas relates that God and men have received their being from the same source because Jesus had preached:

> *"I am not your master…He who will drink from my mouth will become as I am: I myself shall become he, and the things that are hidden will be revealed to him…Let the one who seeks not stop seeking until he finds. When he finds he will be troubled. When he is troubled he will be astonished…the **kingdom (of God) is inside of you, and it is outside of you**. When you come to know yourselves then you will become known and you will realize that you are the sons of the living father… If you bring forth what is within you, what you bring forth will save you. If you do not bring forth what is within you, what you do not bring forth will destroy you".*

The Gospel of Mary says seek the Son of Man within you; look within yourself to find the divine source rather than to Jesus the God Man, just as is expected of a Vedanta practioner. Echoeing renunciation in Vedanta (*neti, neti*), Jesus said: *'The world is a bridge. Pass over it – but do not settle down on it'.* **Jesus believed in reincarnation which was central to the Vedic ideal and which was also widespread in Greece, North Africa, Asia Minor, Anatolia, Egypt and Persia.** The Old Testament speaks of the reincarnation of Elijah and Jesus thought that John the Baptist was reincarnated Elijah. Jesus had proclaimed: *"Verily, verily, I say unto thee, except a man be born again, he cannot see the kingdom of God".* Replying to a question by Nicodemus, Jesus emphasized **"Ye must be born again"**.

Regarding the Universe Jesus replied to Matthew:

> *"I want you to know that he who appeared before the universe in infinity, Self Grown, Self constructed Father, being full of shining light and ineffable, in the beginning, when he decided to have his likeness become a great power, immediately the principle of that Light appeared as Immortal Man …And his consort is the Great Sophia who from the first was destined in him for union by Self-begotten Father, from Immortal Man".*

Like Vedanta, Jesus believed in the purity of thought and speech:

> *"Nothing that originates outside a man can make him unclean by going into him since it doesn't go into his heart…What comes out of man's mouth is what makes him unclean. For it is from within – from the human heart- that evil intentions flow".*

These gospels favor the idea that the **divine is to be discovered on your own** which is **unacceptable to the ordained priest** who controls access to God through the church. Jesus himself certainly never claimed to be God, used to call himself "the Son of Man", and his transformation into a God in human form was not complete until the fourth century. Paul shunted the historical Jesus aside and established Jesus worship as an equivalent of Adonis, of Tammuz, of Attis, or of any other god in the Middle East. In order to compete with these divine rivals, Jesus had to match the miracle for miracle. Virgin birth and resurrection are Pauline inventions, wildly at odds with the 'pure' doctrine preached by James (the brother of Jesus) and the rest of the community in Jerusalem. Paul turned a man into a god and acknowledged that he is not purveying historical Jesus whereas the community in Jerusalem are promulgating "another Jesus" (2 Corinthians 11:3-4) who is now an adversary of Pauline Jesus.

As the **nascent Church** was fighting for its survival 2000 years ago, it organized itself along the feudal model of **serfs and sires** and all but abandoned the Evangelism of the historical Jesus. Dissent was ruthlessly stifled by torture, murder, mutilation, confiscation, excommunication, etc and thought control of the converts was monopolized by the Church hierarchy, employing those very practices and models that it sought to destroy. Arhtus Avalon observed:

> *"The Council of Trent introduced mystic benediction (mantra), incense (dhupa), water (acmana, padya etc), lights (dipa), bells (ghanta), flowers (pushpa), and vestments to aid in the contemplation of the profound mysteries".*

However, the idea of **reincarnation was declared heretical** by the Ecumenical Council of Constantinople in 533 CE so man was no longer responsible for his own spiritual emancipation through right karma. Rather, the access to God now passed through the omnipotent Church hierarchy that alone could save the soul whose fate had already been preordained by God. The human flock was henceforth to be led by the local ecclesiastical shepherd so the slave could worship his master-creator. Second, fearful of the power of the divine goddess, or *Shakti*, so worshipped in Vedanta, Yoga, and around the world, the new religion became an all male monopoly. Paul set the tone:

> *"Let the woman learn in silence with all subjection. But I suffer not a woman to teach, nor to usurp authority over the man, but to be in silence."*

Tertullian in the third century CE continues:

> *"You are the Devil's gateway…the sealer of that forbidden tree…the first deserter of the divine law…. It is not permitted for a woman to speak in Church…to Baptize…to offer the Eucharist, nor to claim for herself a share in any masculine function, least of all in priestly office.*

All mention of Jesus' marital status was removed by the Church decree and Mary Magdalene was turned into a whore. Bishop Clement of Alexandria advised his colleague Theodore to suppress that portion of the Gospel of Mark which speaks of marriage:

> *'…Not all true things are the Truth; nor should that truth which seems true according to human opinions be preferred to the true Truth – that according to the Faith…nor when they*

put forward their falsifications, should one concede that the secret Gospel is by Mark – but should deny it on oath. For not all true things are to be said by all men'.

Human thought was henceforth to be controlled by false premises, eliminations and omissions, decried by the church. As the clergy could not be prosecuted, it freely indulged in sodomy, pedophilia and sexual promiscuity all of which it was supposed to weed out from the society. Such double standards were later on used by people at large to deify Mercantilism, in contrast to the teachings of the historical Jesus.

The second universal religion was born in the early 7th century CE albeit it gave women legal rights of inheritance and divorce all of which were later hijacked by male chauvinism. The Sufi tradition, in Central Asia, shares much in common with Yoga and Vedanta in an external garb of Quranic Islam. The deep *Hum* or *Ho* in *Allaho* reverberates from the heart center and this was revealed to Muhammad as a *mantra* to permit him to go into trances. Finding deeper meanings behind syllabic sounds was followed not only by Sufis but also by the students of Kabbalah. Conservative Islam finally dominated the rebel trends to bring about an intolerant Islam that we know today.

Since both Islam and Christianity called themselves 'true' religions, much blood was spilled over a thousand years of the Christian era in order to decide *the one true God*. As Islam retreated in the 14th century, the Portuguese and the Spanish decimated many races and cultures in the Caribbean and the Pacific, colonized the American continent after depopulating it with their weapons and diseases such as the smallpox, syphilis, tuberculosis, typhoid etc, and established a chain of forts around the world to control the maritime trade. These colonizers even supposed that their God had made them immune to the diseases and that the holocaust was therefore a natural punishment to the heathen for their nonbelief in the one true God. The second phase came two hundred years later when the Dutch, the French and the British attacked the Portuguese in the 16th century to get a piece of the colonial pie, and further decimated peoples and cultures; the 'Magnificient African Cake' was carved out somewhat later. Finally, as it was becoming increasingly difficult to find new peoples and places to exploit, the Western society resorted to exploit its own by the likes of identity theft.

After having raped, tortured, mutilated and murdered in the noble aim of civilizing the heathen, the world wealth was looted as a proof that God had at long last rewarded his chosen people. In the last wave, the cultures and traditions of the decimated heathen are repackaged and even patented as the accomplishments of the master race, while false translations belittled and insulted the historical patrimony of the former subjects. Chakrbarty writes:

"If Buddha's death date can be brought down from 544 to 371 BC then Buddha becomes younger than Pericles (492-420 BC), Socrates (461-399 BC), and Pythagoras. Vaisali, the ancient republic becomes younger than Athens..."

Through such manipulations, the threat that the Vedic past presents to the 'Greek miracle' would be negated by chronology. After having absorbed Vedic-Buddhist knowledge in the sciences and arts, the colonial powers did their best to belittle the past accomplishments of their subject peoples to justify colonialism. To convince themselves of their own superiority, the Aryan invasion hypothesis turned the accomplishments of the ISC peoples into a common Indo-European heritage. In a masterstroke, the achievements of the Vedic people were ascribed to a superior white skinned, blue eyed, Aryan race, coming from somewhere or anywhere, to civilize the dark skinned native who was deemed too inferior to have the capability to realize the marvels in the likes of the ISC. By this simple device, all ancient wisdom now ensued from the Europeans who had come to civilize the Asians in a remote past, though European contributions can be traced no earlier than the 17th-18th centuries of the Christian era. In the worst case scenario, after having decimated the natives in many island nations of the Caribbean and the Pacific, their cultural patrimony was recycled for tourist consumption by the white settlers. Similarly, although the religious fervor of the colonialists all but annihilated many of the priceless traditions of Yoga and Ayurveda, these same colonial masters are now embracing the ancient knowledge and even trying to patent it as their own.

Although still proscribed by the hierarchy of the Patriarchal religions, the 'Yoga in America' study, released by the *Yoga Journal* (2008), shows that Americans spend $5.7 billion a year on yoga classes and products, including equipment, clothing, vacations and media (DVDs, videos, books and magazines). This figure represents an increase of 87% compared to the previous study in 2004. Nearly 6.9% of U.S. adults, or 15.8 million people, practice yoga, but aerobics is practiced by twice as many. Some 6.1%, or nearly 14 million Americans, say that a doctor or therapist has recommended yoga to them. In addition, nearly one half (45%) of all adults agree that yoga would be beneficial if they were undergoing treatment for a medical condition. Yoga Alliance, the world's largest professional organization representing over 20,000 yoga teachers and yoga schools, met on 22 Jan 2009 to streamline their strategy.

Yoga industry exploded when Gucci grabbed headlines with $890 million in sales for yoga mats so that hands and feet don't slide; they run from $10 for vinyl to $50 for natural rubber, and $69 for natural cotton; mat bags start from $10 to $199 for leather. Yoga clothes boast of Zen flare pants and even large, mainstream, apparel makers are putting 'great for yoga' label on everything stretchy. Giants like Ford Motor, Pfizer and Clairol are pursuing well-heeled yogis and Yoga vacations are going strong. The Kripalu Center for Yoga and Health in Lenox, Mass., advertizes a five-day yoga stay from $615 to $1,200 depending on dormitory or luxury room. *Yoga Journal*, founded in 1975, had 310,000 subscribers in 2004, up from 90,000 in 1998, thanks largely to new, big-company advertisers. Beverly Hills yoga master Bikram Choudhury, who put together a sequence of 26 poses in 2002, started sending cease-and-desist orders to studios teaching Bikram yoga, saying they were exploiting his intellectual property. But he incensed his country of birth by getting a U.S. copyright on his style of yoga. India has now put 100 historians and scientists to work, cataloging 1,500 yoga poses recorded in ancient Sanskrit, Urdu and Persian texts, to try to block anyone from patenting the 5,000-year-old discipline of stretching, pranayama and meditation. Although Yoga is denounced by the Anglican Church, in the UK there are just over 10,000 active yoga instructors, teaching between 20,000 and 30,000 yoga classes each week, or an average of 2-3 classes per week catering to 15 students each. This suggests that between 300,000 to 460,000 people currently practice yoga in the UK.

Meanwhile, the New Age Ayurveda has sprung up in the US, UK and Germany. The global pharmaceutical market exceeded US $900 billion in 2008 of which herbal industry accounted for US $62 billion. According to the World Bank, trade in medicinal plants, botanical drug products, and raw materials is growing at an annual growth rate between 5 and 15%. In 2001, US $17.8 billion was spent in the United States on dietary supplements and US $4.2 billion for botanical remedies. In India, botanicals related trade amounts to US $10 billion per annum, with an annual export to the US of $1.1 billion. China's annual herbal drug production is worth US $48 billion per annum; Japan, Hong Kong, Korea and Singapore absorb 66% of China's botanical drugs export. The Western cosmetic industry has started to patent herbal products, after ignoring Ayurvedic knowledge, and is marketing it as original invention. In December 1993, the University of Mississippi Medical Center was granted a patent on the use of turmeric (U.S. patent No. 5,401,504) which was contested by India's Council for Scientific and Industrial Research on the grounds of bio-piracy. After a complex legal battle, the patent was deemed invalid in August 1997 because it was not a novel invention but the knowledge had been derived from Ayurveda. Vandana Shiva, a global campaigner for a fair and honest Intellectual Property Rights system, says patents on herbal products derived from Neem, Amla, Jar Amla, Anar, Salai, Dudhi, Gulmendhi, Bagbherenda, Karela, Erand, Rangoon-kibel, Vilayetishisham and Chamkura also need to be revoked. In 2005, India's National Institute randomly selected 762 U.S. patents that had been granted for medicinal products from plants of which 49% were based on traditional Indian knowledge; about 2,000 patents each year based on India's traditional medicine are taken out somewhere in the world. Seven American and four Japanese firms have filed for patents on formulations of Ashwagandha (*Withania somnifera*) that has been a staple Ayurvedic medicine (chapter 15). The Japanese patent applications wish to use the herb as a skin ointment and for promoting reproductive fertility. The U.S based company Natreon has also obtained a patent for an Ashwagandha extract, while the New England Deaconess Hospital has taken a patent on an Ashwagandha formulation to alleviate symptoms of arthritis. Contrast all this with the Vedic-Buddhist spirit of *krinvantum vishvamaryam*, to do universal good without compensation in return. If the Vedic-Buddhist knowledge were to be patented at the time of discovery, the whole world would be paying royalty to modern India, much as in the past until the colonial era.

Whereas Britain shut down Ayurvedic education in India, all but **decimated some of the Ayurvedic traditions** like the Kayakalpa, and dubbed Tantra Yoga practices in temples as prostitution, it has now accepted Ayurveda as part of its National Health Service. An agreement signed by Indian High Commission will permit relative quacks in the UK to become licensed Ayurveda practitioners, after just 1,600 hours of training, whereas it requires up to six years in India. Gopi Warrier, chairman of the privately-run British Ayurvedic Medical Council, and owner of the Ayurveda Company of Great Britain, remarks:

> *"It is my karma to protect Ayurveda and prevent toddy being marketed as champagne. I believe India should have at least a 60 per cent share of the huge market in Ayurveda therapy and products. But the Indian government appears to have gone to sleep and Indian officials here are to blame that Britain plans to introduce a lamentably short Ayurveda course of study before one can say one is qualified".*

Although Yoga and Ayurveda were meant to lead the individual to acquire a sattvic mind, most yoga adepts in the West have all but ignored the spiritual aspects, concentrating only on the physical benefits for ever greater indulgence in 'good life' (ethylism, toxicomania and promiscuity). As there is no professional follow-up, with passing years many yoga teachers gain weight, are unable to enter into demanding yoga postures, and to maintain them for any more than just a few seconds. Many yoga teachers neither understand nor are able to pronounce even simple Sanskrit words like Pranayama. Although Ayurvedic texts prescribe strict procedures for the collection of medicinal plants from their natural habitats (Chapter 15), owners of herb shops in the west are fooling people into purchasing plants grown under artificial conditions in green houses. These cultivated herbs are largely devoid of active ingredients that are synthesized only under the right combination of soil, sun, humidity, and so forth. Worse still, even artificial products are being marketed under the title Aromatherapy although they cannot possibly impart the benefits of essential oils and other active ingredients in natural products, and can even be harmful. Meanwhile, massage parlors in SE-Asia are offering the likes of 'Indian head massage' and 'ShiroAbhyanga' without having the vaguest notion about marmas, nadis or acupressure. The sole emphasis is mercantilism by any and all means, while the spiritual message of their own faith has been all but ignored; Jesus had said: '*It is easier for a camel to pass through the eye of a needle, than for a rich man to enter the kingdom of God*'. The two tenets of the Kingdom of God in the Bible were: universal peace and uplift of the poor. A recent analysis by Hughes has shown that the US not only thrives by accelerating, not defusing, conflicts around the world, it spends only 0.2% of the GNP for social services to uplift the poor, and a majority of the citizens do not have access to proper medical services. In fact, the rich and privileged jealously temper all attempts for reform in this direction because wealth is believed to represent special favor by God, in contrast to the teachings ascribed to the historical Jesus. Muslims, too, seem to have gone against their initial fury and are now not only using Sanskrit names to market their products, but also manufacturing Ayurvedic products without much knowledge about the subject.

Paradoxically, while the West has turned away from the frigid sterility of the middle ages and the vanity of the Victorian era, people and politicians of modern India look to the west for inspiration and despise their own ancient patrimony. The current education in India follows the British tradition whose purpose it was to plant an inferiority complex in the mind of its colonial subjects and make them look to the west for inspiration (Chapter 1). Post-independent India was particularly unfortunate in having British-oriented people like Gandhi and Nehru as its leaders. While M.K. Gandhi preached nonviolence for India, he actively recruited for the military duty to help the British war effort. Although denied membership in an exclusive British only club in India, Nehru remained loyal to the British until his death and even led a promiscuous life that was the hallmark of Victorian England. Like the British, **Nehru** not only condemned Tantra Yoga but also prominently remarked that he was: "*…proud to be reared up as an Islamist, an Englishman by education, and Hindu by accident*". In a letter to President Dr Rajendra Prasad (Nov 17, 1953) **Nehru** even managed to reverse the definition of tolerance: "*The Hindu is certainly not tolerant and is certainly more narrow minded than almost any person in any other country* *except the Jews"*. The mission of the British educational policy under Macaulay (Chapter 1) has thus come to full fruitition by perpetuating the feigned inferiority of their ancient colonial subjects.

How we see ourselves is shaped by the history we absorb as it fires our imagination and curiosity. Rulers throughout history have recognized that the control of the past is required to master the present to consolidate power. There was one British soldier for every 4000 Indians and an Englishman was lucid: *had all the Indians chosen to spit at the same moment his countrymen would have drowned.* Field Marshal Lord Roberts summarized the British rule:

> *"It is this consciousness of the inherent superiority of the European which has won us India. However well educated and clever a native may be and however brave he may have proved himself, I believe that no rank which we can bestow upon him would cause `him to be considered an equal by the British officer"*.

There is no greater humiliation than mental servitude because this voluntarily reduces the individual to slavery. In the Phrenology of Spirit (1807 CE), Hegel developed the Master-Slave Dialectic where the slave had accepted its role as the lesser of the two and saw itself only as a slave in the state of *Thinghood* whose job was to recognize the master. While a rebellious spirit freed the world of physical fetters of the colonial era, an enslaved mind has assured voluntary perpetuation of the myth of racial inferiority invented by the masters to control the slaves. Love for everything foreign, adoration for white skin, and criticism of everything indigenous, are hallmarks of contemporary India. The death bed message of Tagore was rife with premonition:

> *"I had at one time believed that the springs of civilization would issue out of the heart of Europe. But today when I am about to quit the world that faith has gone bankrupt altogether...How I wish I could embrace my India and shield her from all the insults heaped upon her. The sahibs kick us all the time, yet we do not leave their doorstep. Where they do not let us enter with our shoes on, we leave our shoes behind. Where they do not let us enter with our heads high we enter with bowed heads. Where we are denied admittance as Indians, we go in guise of Englishmen. They do not want us and yet we find excuses, we cringe and cower and at the slightest opportunity we try to seek their company isolating ourselves from our countrymen and even joining them in the abuse of the nation"*.

Jai Bharata

18.
Bibliography

Acharya, Deepak and Shrivastava, Anshu, Indigenous Herbal Medicines: Tribal Formulations and Traditional Herbal Practices, Aavishkar Publishers, Jaipur, 2008.

Ahir, D. C., Buddhism Declined in India: How and Why? B. R. Publishing, ND, 2005.

Alan, Keith Tillotson, Nai-shing Hu, Tillotson, Abel, Robert, The One Earth Herbal Sourcebook: Everything You Need to Know About Chinese, Western, and Ayurvedic Herbal Treatments, Kensington press, 2001.

Aldridge, David, Music Therapy in Dementia Care, Jessica Kingsley, London, 2000.

Ali, M., A brief history of Indian alchemy covering pre-Vedic to Vedic and Ayurvedic periods (circa 400 BC-800 AD), Bulletin Indian Institute for History of Medicine., Hyderabad, 23: 151-166, 1993.

Amadea, Morningstar and Desai, Urmila, The Ayurvedic Cookbook, Motilala Barsidas, ND, 2005.

Anant, Sadashiv Altekar, Education in Ancient India, Nand Kishore and Brothers, Varanasi, 1965.

Andrew, Biel and Robin, Dorn, Trail Guide to The Body. Books of Discovery, Boulder, CO, 2005.

Armstrong, Karen, A History of God, Ballantine Books, NY, 1993.

Asher, Catherine, B. and Talbot, Cynthia, India Before Europe, Cambridge, 2006.

Atmananda, Swami, All You Wanted to Know about Tantra Yoga, New Dawn, ND, 2002.

Avalon, Arthur, Sakti and Sakta, Ganesh and Co., 1918.

Avalon, Arthur, Tantra of the Great Liberation - Mahanirvana Tantra, Dover publications, NY, 1972.

Avalon, Arthur, The Principles of Tantra, London, 1914-1916.

Aung, Steven, Lee, K.H., Mathew H.M., Music, Sounds, Medicine, and Meditation: An Integrative Approach to the Healing Arts, Alternative and Complementary Therapies, 10: 266-270, 2004.

Ayurved ki Nai Shodha, Electro-tridosha-graphy, Mystic India, ND, January 2006.

Bachorowski, J.A., Smoski, M.J. and Owren, M.J., The Acoustic Features of Human Laughter. Journal Acoustical Society of America 110: 1581, 2001.

Baginski, B. J.,Sharamon, S., Reiki: Universal Life Energy, Life Rhythm, 1988.

Bakhru, H. K., Nature Cure, Jaico Publishing, Mumbai, 2006.

Balachandran, Premalatha, Govindarajan, Rajgopal, Ayurvedic Drug Discovery, Information Healthcare, 2: 1631-1652, 2007.

Barrett, Dierdre, The Power of Hypnosis, Psychology Today. Jan/Feb 2001.

Berzin, Alexander. The Four Indian Buddhist Tenet Systems Regarding Illusion: A Practical Approach. Berlin, 2002.

Bhattacharyya, N. N. History of the Tantric Religion. Manohar Lal Banarsidas, ND, 1999.

Bogard, M., Laughter and its Effects on Groups, Bullish Press, NY, 2008.

Boso, M., Politi, P., Barale, F., Enzo, E., Neurophysiology and Neurobiology of the Musical Experience. Functional Neurol., 21: 87–91 2006.

Bynum, William, The History of Medicine, Oxford, NY, 2008.

Hermann, Kulke and Dietmar, Rothermund, A History of India, Routledge, 2004.

Buhnemann, Gudrun, The Worship of Mahaga apati According to the Nityotsava, Kant Publications, 2003.

Carl, Edwin Lindgren, Capturing the Aura, Blue Dolphin, Nevada, 2005.

Cartwright, Steven, On the nature of Homeopathy, The Homeopath, 62: 599-601, 1996.

Cathell, D. W., Cathell W.T., Book on the Physician Himself, FA Davis & Co., Philadelphia, 1911.

Chaplin, Dorothy, Matter, Myth and Spirit, or Keltic and Hindu Links, Scot Rider & Co., London, UK, 1935.

Chopra, R. N., Chopra, I. C., Handa, K. L., Kapur, L. D. in Chopra's indigenous drugs of India. Dhur and Sons, Calcutta, 1958.

Chopra, R. N., Nayar, S. L. and Chopra, I. C.,Glossary of Indian Medicinal plants. CSIR, ND, 1992.

McMohan, Christopher, Indian attars, International Journal of Aromatherapy, 7, 10-13, 1996.

Cohn-Haft, Louis, The Public Physicians of Ancient Greece, Northampton, Massachusetts, 1956

Conrad, Lawrence I., Neve, Michael, Nutton, Vivian, Porter, Roy, Wear, Andrew. The Western Medical Tradition: 800 BC to AD 1180, Cambridge, 1995.

Crussi, Gonzalez F., A Short History of Medicine, Random House, NY, 2007.

Cumston, Charles Greene, An Introduction to the History of Medicine, Alfred A Knopf, NY, 1926.

Dutt, Sukumar, Buddhist Monks And Monasteries Of India: Their History and Contribution To Indian Culture, Allen and Unwin, London, 1962.

Diemer, Deedre, The ABC's of Chakra Therapy, Motilal Banarsidas, ND, 2000.

Emmerick, Ronald E., The Siddhasara of Ravigupta, Steiner Verlag, 1980.

Falk, H., Soma I and II. Bulletin of the School of Oriental and African Studies, 52: 77-90,1989.

Feurstein, George, Kak, Subhash, Frawley, David, In Search of the Cradle of Civilization, Quest Books, Illinois, 1995.

Finegold, Leonard, Magnet Therapy, British Medical Journal, 332: 4, 2006.

Frank, John Ninivaggi, An Elementary Textbook of Ayurveda: Medicine with a Six Thousand Year Old Tradition, International Universities Press, Madison, WI, 2001.

Frawley, David, Yoga and Ayurveda: Self-Healing and Self-Realization, Lotus Press, NM, 2000.

Frawley, David, Ranade, Subhash and Lele, Avinash, Ayurveda and Marma Therapy, Lotus Press, NM, 2003.

Frawley, David and Vasant Lad, The Yoga of Herbs: An Ayurvedic Guide to Herbal Medicine, Lotus Press, Santa Fe, NM, 1986.

Frawley, David, Ayurvedic Healing: A Comprehensive Guide, Motilal Banarsidas, ND, 1997.

Fried, I., Wilson, C.L., MacDonald, K.A. and Behnke E.J., Electric Current Stimulates Laughter. Nature, 391:650, 1998.

Frost, Gavin and Frost,Yvonne, Tantric Yoga, Motilal Banarsidas, ND,1994.

Garraty, John, A., Gay, Peter (eds) The Columbia History of the World, Harper and Row, NY, 1985.

Garrisson, T., An Introduction to the History of medicine, Saunders, Philadelphia, 1929.

Gertrude, Emerson, The Story of Early Indian Civilization, Orient Longmans, 1964.

Gode, P. K., Studies in the History of Indian Cosmetics and Perfumery: Notes on the history of the rose, rose-water and attar of roses—between BC 500 and AD 1850, New Indian Antiquary 8, 107-119, 1961.

Goel, V., Dolan, R. J., The Functional Anatomy of Humor: Segregating Cognitive and Affective Components. Nature Neuroscience 3: 237-238, 2001.

Greig, John, Young, Thomson, The Psychology of Comedy and Laughter, Dodd Mead and company, NY, 1923.

Gupta, S. P., The Indus-Saraswati Civilization, Pratibha Prakashan, ND, 1996.

Guthrie, W. K. C., A History of Greek Philosophy, Volume I: The earlier Presocratics and the Pythagoreans. Cambridge, NY, 1962.

Hanser S. B. and Thompson L.W., Effects of a Music Therapy Strategy on Depressed Older Adults, J Gerontol. 49: 265–269, 1994.

Harper, Katherine Anne and Robert, Brown, L. (eds), The Roots of Tantra. State U New York Press, 2002.

Henderson, Tony, Disorderly Women in Eighteenth Century London, Person Educational Ltd, UK, 1999.

Hermann, Kulke and Dietmar, Rothermund, A History of India, Routledge, 2004.

Herz, R. S., Aromatherapy Facts and Fiction: a Scientific Analysis, Int. J. Neurosci, 119: 263-290, 2009.

Hoernle, A. F. Rudolf (ed), The Bower Manuscript; Facsimile Leaves, Nagari Transcript, Romanised Transliteration and English Translation with Notes, Calcutta, 1893-1912, Aditya Prakashan, ND, 1987..

Holland, Alex, Voices of Qi, An Introductory Guide to Traditional Chinese Medicine, North Atlantic Books, 2000.

Homewood, A.E., The Neurodynamics of the Vertebral Subluxation, Valkyrie Press, 1979.

Hopkins, Jeffrey, Meditation on Emptiness, Wisdom Publications, 1996.

Hosak, Mark, Luebeck, Walter, Big Book of Reiki Symbols, Lotus Press, 2006.

Huffman, M.A., Animal Self-Medication and Ethno-Medicine: Exploration and Exploitation of the Medicinal Properties of Plants, Proc. Nutr. Soc., 62, 371–81, 2003.

Hughes, Richard, T., Christian America and the Kingdom of God, U. Illinois press, IL, 2009.

Hutchings, M.R., Athanasiadou, S., Kyriazakis. I. and Gordon, I.J., Can Animals Use Foraging Behavior to Combat Parasites?. Proc. Nutr. Soc., 62: 361-370, 2003.

Igor, Krichtafovitch, Humor Theory. The Formulae of Laughter, Outskits press, 2006.

Jacquart, Danielle, Islamic Pharmacology in the Middle Ages: Theories and Substance, European Review,16: 219–227, 2008.

Jeong S., Kim M.T., Effects of a Theory-Driven Music and Movement Program for Stroke Survivors in a Community Setting. Appl. Nurs. Res., 20: 125–131, 2007.

Jones, W. H. S. Philosophy and Medicine in Ancient Greece, Johns Hopkins, Baltimore, 1946.

Joshi, Sunil, Ayurveda and Panchakarma, Motilal Banarsidas, ND, 1998.

Kacera, Walter, Ayurvedic Tongue Diagnosis, Lotus Press, Twin Lakes, WI, 2006.

Kapoor, J.N., Attars of India - A Unique Aroma, Perfumer and Flavorist, 1991.

Kawakami, K., Takai-Kawakami K., Tomohaga, M., Siuzuki, J., Okai, T., Origins of Smile and Laughter: A preliminary study, Early Human Development 82: 61-66, 2006.

Kersten, Holger, Jesus Lived in India, Element Books Ltd., UK,1994.

Kenoyer, J. M., From Summer to Meluhaa, Prehistory Press, Madison, 1994.

Kenoyer, Jonathan, Uncovering the Keys to Lost Indus Cities. Scientific American, July 2003.

Kenoyer, Jonathan, Ancient Cities of the Indus Valley Civilization, Oxford, NY, 1998.

Kilner, Walter J., The Human Aura, Citadel Press, NY, 1965,

Kilner, Walter J., The Aura, S. Weiser, NY, 1973.

Kim, S. J., The Effects of Music on Pain Perception of Stroke Patients During Upper Extremity Joint Exercises. J. Music Therapy. 42: 81-92, 2005.

Kinjavadekara, R.S., Astanga Samgraha, Uppal Publishing House, ND, 1998.

Knapp, Stephen, Proof of Vedic Culture's Global Existence, Booksurge, Charleston, SC, 2000.

Knapp, Stephen, Crimes Against India and the Need to Protect its Ancient Vedic Tradition: 1000 Years of Attack Against Hinduism and what to do about it. iUniverse.com 2009.

Koch C., Reichling J., Schneele J., Schnitzler, P., Inhibitory effect of essential oils against herpes simplex virus type 2. Phytomedicine, 15, 71-78, 2008.

Krishnamurthy R., Perfumery in Ancient India, Indian J. Hist. Sci., 22, 71-79, 1987.

Lad, Vasant, Ayurveda, The Science of Self-Healing, Motilal Banarsidas, New Delhi, 1994.

Lai, P.K., Antimicrobial and Chemopreventive Properties of Herbs and Spices. Curr. Med. Chem., 1451-1460, 2004.

LaRoche, Dain, and Declan A. J., Effects of Stretching on Passive Muscle Tension and Response to Eccentric Exercise, American Journal of Sports Medicine 34: 1000-1007, 2006.

Lennox, James, Aristotle's Biology, Stanford Encyclopedia of Philosophy, 2006.

Lichtheim, Miriam, Ancient Egyptian Literature, London, 1975.

Longrigg, James, Greek Rational Medicine: Philosophy and Medicine from Alcmæon to the Alexandrians, Routledge, 1993.

Luebeck, Walter, The Complete Reiki Handbook. Motilal Banarsidas, ND,1998.

Luebeck, Walter, Petter, F. A., Rand, W.L., Spirit of Reiki, Lotus Press, 2004.

MacDonald, C., A Chuckle a Day Keeps the Doctor Away: Therapeutic Humor and Laughter, Journal of Psychosocial Nursing and Mental Health Services 42:18-25, 2004.

Maciocia, Giovanni, The Foundations of Chinese Medicine: A Comprehensive Text for Acupuncturists and Herbalists, Churchill Livingstone, 1997.

Maenthaisong R, Chaiyakunapruk N, Niruntraporn S. et al. The efficacy of Aloe Vera for Burn Wound Healing: a Systematic Review. Burns. 33:713-718, 2007.

Magee, W.L., Davidson, J.W., The effect of Music Therapy on Mood States in Neurological Patients: A Pilot Study, J. Music Therapy 39: 20-29, 2002.

Mahdihassan, S. Parisrut, The Earliest Distilled Liquor of Vedic times about 1500 BC. Indian J. His. Sci., 16, 223-229, 1981.

Major, Arthur, Powell, E., The Etheric Double and Allied Phenomena, Quest Books, Il., 1969.

Marcus, Steven, The Other Victorians, Basic Books Inc., NY, 1964.

Marteinson, Peter, On the Problem of the Comic: A Philosophical Study on the Origins of Laughter, Legas Press, Ottawa, 2006.

McEvilley, Thomas, The Shape of Ancient Thought, Allworth Press, NY, 2002.

Milius, S., Don't Look Now, but is that Dog Laughing? Science News 160, 55, 2001.

Morningstar, Amadea, and Desai, Urmila, The Ayurvedic Cook Book, Motilal Banarsidas, ND, 2005

Mukhopadhyaya, Girindranath, The surgical Instrument of the Hindus, with a Comparative Study of the Surgical Instruments of the Greek, Roman, Arab and the Modern European surgeons, New Bharatiya Book Corporation, Calcutta, 2000.

Muktibodhananda, Swami, Hatha Yoga Pradipika, Munger, India, 1993.

Multhauf, Robert, P. and Gilbert, Robert Andrew, Alchemy. Encyclopædia Britannica, 2008.

Murthy K.R.S., Sarangadhara Samhita of Pt.Sarangadharacharya, Varanasi, 1987.

Murthy K.R.S., Bhavaprakasa of Bhavamisra, Madhya and Uttara Khanda, Krishnadas Academy, Varanasi, 2001.

Nayak, S., Wheeler, B. L., Shiflett, S.C., Agostinelli, S., Effect of Music Therapy on Mood and Social Interaction Among Individuals with Acute Traumatic Brain Injury and Stroke. Rehabilitation Psychology 45: 274-283, 2000.

Nehru, J.L., The Discovery of India, Oxford, ND, 1985.

Ni, Mao-Shing, The Yellow Emperor's Classic of Medicine: A New Translation of the Neijing Suwen with Commentary, Shambhala, 1995.

Norbu, Chogyal Namkhai, The Crystal and The Way of Light: Sutra, Tantra and Dzogchen, Snow Lion Publications, 1999.

O'Flaherty, Wendy Doniger, The post-Vedic history of the Soma plant. In R. Gordon Wasson (ed) Soma: divine mushroom of immortality, Harcourt, Brace Janovitch, 1971.

Omprakash, Yemul, India Where Attars Originated, India Perspectives, 2004.

Oon, Kim, India's Religious Quest, Young Golden Gate Publishing Co.,1976.

Oliver, Klatt, Reiki Systems of the World, Lotus Press, 2007.

Oscar Bagnall, The Origin and Properties of the Human Aura, 1937.

Osler, William, The Evolution of Modern medicine, Yale U Press, New Haven, 1921.

Pain, Stephanie,The Pharaohs' Pharmacists, New Scientist, pp 41- 43. 15 December, 2007.

Panksepp, J. and Burgdorf, J., Laughing Rats and the Evolutionary Antecedents of Human Joy. Physiology and Behavior 79: 533-547, 2003.

Pareti, Luigi, The Ancient World, Parts I-III, UNESCO, Allan and Unwin, London, 1965.

Petter, F. A., Yamaguchi, T., and Hayashi, C., Hayashi Reiki Manual: Traditional Japanese Healing Techniques from the Founder of the Western Reiki System, Lotus Press, 2004.

Philippa, Levine, Prostitution, Race and Politics, Routledge, NY, 2003.

Pickering, Judith, Being in Love, Routledge, NY, 2008.

Pilates, Joseph, H., Pilates: Return to Life through Contrology, Christopher Publishing House, 1960.

Pittler, Max H., Brown, E. M., Ernst, E., Static Magnets for Reducing Pain: Systematic Review and Meta-Analysis of Randomized Trials, Canadian Med. Assoc. J., 177: 7, 2007.

Plinio Prioreschi, A History of Medicine, Horatius Print, 1996.

Polk, Charles, Elliot Postow, Handbook of Biological Effects of Electromagnetic Fields, CRC Press, 1996.

Pollock, Sheldon, Forms of Knowledge in Early Modern Asia: Explorations in the Intellectural History of India and Tibet. Amazon.com, 2011.

Powicke, F. M. and Emden, A. B., Rashdall's Medieval Universities, Clarendon Press, Oxford, 1936.

Prabhakar, Chatterjee, Ras Chikitsa, Chowkhamba, Banaras, 1956.

Priyavrat Sharma and Karambekar, V.W., The Atharvaveda and the Ayurveda, Nagpur 1961.

Provine, R. R., Laughter, American Scientist, 84: 38-45, 1996.

Possehl,Gregory L., The Indus Civilization, Brown and Littlefield, Latham, MD, 2002.

Possehl, Gregory L. The Indus Writing System, U. Penn., Philadelphia, PA, 1996.

Possehl, Gregory, L. The Ancient Cities of the Indus, Vikas, New Delhi, 1979.

Puri, H.S., Rasayan: Ayurvedic Herbs of Rejuvenation and Longevity, Taylor and Francis, London, 2003.

Puri, H.S., Ayurvedic Minerals, Gems and Animal Products for Longevity and Rejuvenation. India Book Store, ND, 2006.

Qureshi, Samina, Legacy of the Indus, Weatherhill, NY, 1974.

Radha, Swami Sivananda, Kundalini Yoga, Motilal Banarsidas, ND,1992.

Radha, Kumud Mookerji, Ancient Indian Education: Brahmanical and Buddhist, Motilal Banarsidass, New Delhi, 1989.

Radha, Kumud Mookerji, Chandragupta Maurya and His Times. Motilal Banarsidass, ND, 1989.

Ray, Priyadaranjan and Gupta, Hirendra Nath, Charaka Samhita, Indian National Science Academy, ND, 1980.

Ray, Priyadaranjan, Gupta, Hirendra Nath and Roy, Mira. Sushuruta Samhita. Indian National Science Academy, ND, 1980.

Rele, V. G., The Vedic Gods as Figures of Biology, Taraporevala and Sons, Bombay, 1931.

Rhyner, Hans, H., Ayurveda, The Gentle Health System, Motilal Banarsidas, ND, 1998.

Ranade, Subhash and Frawley, David, Natural Healing through Ayurveda, Motilal Banarsidas, 1999.

Rege, N.N, Thatte, U.M, Dahanukar, S.A., Adaptogenic properties of six rasayan herbs used in Ayurvedic medicine. Phytother. Res.,13: 275-291, 1999.

Rene, Grousset, In the Footsteps of the Buddha, Orion Press. NY, 1971.

Renfrew, Colin, Before Civilization: The Radiocarbon Revolution and Prehistoric Europe, Penguin, 1990.

Ringdal, Johan, Nils, Love for Sale, A World History of Prostitution, Grove Press, NY, 2004.

Rousselle, Aline, Porneia, Blackwell, 1988.

Sah, Ram Lal, Joshi, Binod Kumar and Joshi, Geeta, Vedic Health Care System, New Age Books, ND, 2002.

Saraswati, Swami Satyananda, Sure Ways to Self Realization. Yoga Publications Trust, 2000.

Sarton, A., History of Science, W.W. Norton and Company, 1952.

Sastri, Subbaraya, Discovery of Ayurveda, Nagarjun, 1976.

Scott, David, Buddhism and Islam: Past to Present Encounters and Interfaith Lessons., Numen, 42: 141,-155, 1995.

Scott, Gerson, Ayurvedic Guide to Diet and Weight Loss, Lotus Press, Twin Lakes, Wisconsin, 2002.

Schneider, S., Schönle, P.W., Altenmüller, E., Munte, T. F., Using Musical Instruments to Improve Motor Skill Recovery Following a Stroke. J. Neurol., 254: 1339–1346, 2007.

Segal, N.A., Hein, J., Basford. J.R., The Effects of Pilates Training on Flexibility and Body Composition: an Observational Study, Arch. Phys. Med. Rehabil., 85:1977–1981, 2004.

SenGupta, Vinod Lal, Ayurveda Vijnanam, Calcutta, 1929.

Sharma P.V., Chakradatta: a Treatise on Principles and Practices of Ayurvedic Medicine, Vedam Books International, ND, 1998.

Singhal, G.D.and Patterson, T.J.S. Synopsis of Ayurveda, Based on a Translation of Susuruta Samhita, Oxford, ND, 1993.

Spink, M. S. and Lewis, G. L. (eds). Albucasis on Surgery and Instruments, Wellcome Trust, UK, 1973.

Stalker, Douglas, Glymour, Clark, Examining Holistic Medicine, Prometheus, Buffalo, NY, 1985.

Stanmore, Tia, The Pilates Back Book: Head, Neck, Back, and Shoulder Pain With Easy Pilates Stretches, Fair Winds Press, Gloucester, MA, 2004.

Swami, Rama, Ballentine, Rudolph, Hymes, Alan, Science of Breath, Himalayan International Institute, Honesdale, Pennsylvania, 1979.

Swami, Veda Bharati, Mantra and Meditation, Himalayan International Institute, Honesdale, Pennsylvania, 1981.

Swami, Vishnu Devananda, Meditation and Mantras, Motilal Banarsidas, ND, 1978.

Talwar, N., Crawford, Mike J., Maratos, Anna, Nur, Ula, McDermott, Orii, Procter, Simon, Music Therapy for in-Patients with Schizophrenia: Exploratory Randomised Controlled Trial, Brit. J. Psychiatry, 189: 405–409, 2006.

Tapsell, L.C., Health Benefits of Herbs and Spices: the Past, the Present, the Future. Med. J. Aust., 1, 2006.

Taylor, Timothy, The Prehistory of Sex, Bantam, NY, 1996.

Trevor, Fisher, Prostitution and the Victorians, St. Martins Press, NY, 1997.

Tschanz, David, W., Arab Roots of European Medicine, Heart Views, 2003.

Tuet, R.W.K. and Lam, L.C.W., A preliminary study of the effects of music therapy on agitation in Chinese patients with dementia, Hong Kong Journal of Psychiatry, Volume 16, 2006.

Usui, M., Petter, F. A., Original Reiki Handbook of Dr. Mikao Usui, Lotus Press, 2003.

Urban, Hugh, Tantra: Sex, Secrecy, Politics, and Power in the Study of Religions, University of California Press, 2003.

Useful Technology to detect the effects of Panchakarma in Human body, ETG, Scientific Journal of Panchakarma, Ujjain, MP, July 2005.

Verma, Vinod, Patanjali and Ayurvedic Yoga, Motilala Banarsidas, ND, 2001.

Verma, Vinod, Stress-free work with Yoga and Ayurveda, New Age Books, 2003.

Vink, A., Music and emotion: Living apart together: A relationship between music psychology and music therapy. Nordic Journal of Music Therapy. 10: 144-158, 2001.

Vishnu Devananda, Swami, Hatha Yoga, Pradipika, Motilal Banarsidas, ND, 1999.

Vickers, Andrew and Zollman, Catherine, Clinical review. ABC of complementary medicine. Hypnosis and relaxation therapies, British Medical Journal, 319:1346-1349, 1999.

Vogler, B.K., Ernst, E., Aloe vera: a Systematic Review of its Clinical Effectiveness, Br. J. Gen. Prac., 49: 823-828,1999.

Wangyal, RinpocheTenzin and Dahlby, Mark, The Tibetan Yogas of Dream and Sleep, Lion Publications, NY, 1998.

Weerapong, Pornratshanee, Patria A. Hume, Gregory S. Kolt, Stretching: Mechanisms and Benefits for Sports Performance and Injury Prevention Physical Therapy Reviews 9:189-206, 2004.

Wheeler, Mortimer, Civilizations of the Indus Valley and Beyond, McGraw Hill, NY, 1965.

Whipple, Jennifer, Music in Intervention for Children and Adolescents with Autism: A Meta-Analysis., Journal of Music Therapy, 41: 90–106, 2004.

White, David Gordon (ed) Tantra in Practice, Princeton University Press, 2000.

White, David Gordon, Kiss of the Yogini : "Tantric Sex" in its South Asian Contexts. U. Chicago Press, 2003.

Wigram, Tony, A Method of Music Therapy Assessment for the Diagnosis of Autism and Communication Disorders in Children. Music Therapy Perspectives, 18: 13–22, 2002.

Winston, David and Maimes, Steven. Adaptogens: Herbs for Strength, Stamina, and Stress Relief, Healing Arts Press, 2007.

Wolpert, Stanley, A New History of India, Oxford, 2004.

Wujastyk, Dominik, Ravigupta and Vagbhata, Bulletin of the School of Oriental and African Studies, 48: 74-78, 1985.

Wujastyk, Dominik, The Roots of Ayurveda, Penguin, India, 1998.

Yeshe, Lama Thubten, Introduction to Tantra: The Transformation of Desire, Wisdom Publications, Boston, 2001.

Zysk, Kenneth, G., Medicine in the Veda, Motilal Banarsidas, ND, 1996.

Zysk, Kenneth, G., Asceticism and Healing in Ancient India: Medicine in the Buddhist Monastery, Motilal Banarsidas, ND, 1998.

19.

Abbreviated Index

CPSIA information can be obtained
at www.ICGtesting.com
Printed in the USA
BVOW09s0527031217
501445BV00008BA/249/P